Take Control of Your Period

The Well-Timed Period:
From Quality-of-Life to
Cancer Prevention

* * *

DIANA KROI, M.D.

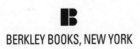

BERKLEY BOOKS, NEW YORK

Most Berkley Books are available at special quantity discounts for bulk purchases for sales promotions premiums, fundraising, or educational use. Special book, or book excerpts, can also be created to fit specific needs. For details, write: Special Markets, The Berkley Publishing Group, 375 Hudson Street, New York, New York 10014.

THE BERKLEY PUBLISHING GROUP
Published by the Penguin Group
Penguin Group (USA) Inc.
375 Hudson Street, New York, New York 10014, USA
Penguin Group (Canada), 10 Alcorn Avenue, Toronto, Ontario M4V 3B2, Canada
(a division of Pearson Penguin Canada Inc.)
Penguin Books Ltd., 80 Strand, London WC2R 0RL, England
Penguin Group Ireland, 25 St. Stephen's Green, Dublin 2, Ireland (a division of Penguin Books Ltd.)
Penguin Group (Australia), 250 Camberwell Road, Camberwell, Victoria 3124, Australia
(a division of Pearson Australia Group Pty. Ltd.)
Penguin Books India Pvt. Ltd., 11 Community Centre, Panchsheel Park, New Delhi—110 017, India
Penguin Group (NZ), Cnr. Airborne and Rosedale Roads, Albany, Auckland 1310, New Zealand
(a division of Pearson New Zealand Ltd.)
Penguin Books (South Africa) (Pty.) Ltd., 24 Sturdee Avenue, Rosebank, Johannesburg 2196, South Africa

Penguin Books Ltd., Registered Offices: 80 Strand, London WC2R 0RL, England

This book is an original publication of The Berkley Publishing Group.

Neither the publisher nor the author is engaged in rendering professional advice or services to the individual reader. The ideas, procedures, and suggestions contained in this book are not intended as a substitute for consulting with your physician. All matters regarding your health require medical supervision. Further, this book may mention uses of regimens not approved by the FDA or recommended by the manufacturer. Neither the author nor the publisher shall be liable or responsible for any loss or damage allegedly arising from any information or suggestion in this book.

All examples are based on actual encounters; however, the names and identifiable details have been changed to protect the patients' privacy.

PRINTING HISTORY
Berkley trade paperback edition / October 2004
Berkley trade paperback ISBN: 0-425-19949-5

Library of Congress Cataloging-in-Publication Data

Kroi, Diana.
    Take control of your period / Diana Kroi.—Berkley trade pbk. ed.
        p. cm.
    Includes bibliographical references.
    ISBN 0-425-19949-5
        1. Menstruation—Prevention. 2. Contraceptive drugs—Physiological effect.
    3. Menstruation—Psychological aspects. I. Title.

    QP263.K765 2004
    618.1'72—dc22   2004055062

PRINTED IN THE UNITED STATES OF AMERICA

10   9   8   7   6   5   4   3   2   1

This book is dedicated to all the women of the world
and to the men who love and respect them.

Acknowledgements

To my family and friends (you know who you are): thank you for your support and your patience.

To all my patients: thank you for the privilege of allowing me to be your doctor. To all my professors and colleagues: thank you for the opportunity to learn, do, and teach.

Finally, to each and every one of the individuals involved with bringing this book to light—Felicia Eth, Denise Silvestro, Katie Day, Jennifer Anderson, to name but a few: I thank you for your vision, trust, and guidance.

Contents

Introduction

"I can't believe I'm getting my period today, of all days!" Does this sound familiar to you? Let's face it—if you're a woman, chances are you've uttered those words at some time in your life.

For thirty-five years of their lives, most women have a monthly menstrual period. That can add up to over 450 periods in a lifetime. That's 450 chances that your period may impact your health, your school and work pursuits, your personal life, the lives of your family and loved ones, or even society at large. Surprisingly, many of the 60 million women of menstruating age in the United States think that there's little they can do to manage or minimize the impact of their periods. Luckily, nothing could be further from the truth. You, in consultation with your physician, can manage your period. Period control, or menstrual management, is a reality and it has been around for almost half a century. Talk about a "best kept secret"!

Understanding the basics of your period and menstrual management will help you decide if the technique is right for you. It will also give you the power to control your period, from occasionally scheduling when your period begins to reducing the number of yearly periods from thirteen to as few as four.

If, at this point, you're asking yourself, "What can menstrual management do for *me*?" it may help to think about the times when your period has interfered with your life, everything from routine daily tasks to major life events.

For example, think back to your high school prom. For millions of women, that was the exact day they got their period. For some, cramping marred a once-in-a-lifetime event. Or perhaps you're in college, ready to venture on your first spring break, for a week of "fun in the sun." Better leave enough room in your luggage for tampons—you never know. And, when you spend countless months planning the perfect wedding and honeymoon, don't forget to pencil in your menstrual period.

But periods don't affect just special events; they disrupt people's daily lives. They affect teachers who are always present, patient, and available for their students, despite tremendous personal discomfort from periods. They affect nurses, who once a month may be bleeding more than their patients. They affect the stay-at-home mom who has to take care of a sick family, in spite of monthly cramps. They can be a life-threatening problem for the soldier who has to defend her country and the policewoman who is always on duty and ready to act, period or no period. Even more seriously, millions of women are plagued by period-related health problems like anemia, migraine headaches, endometriosis, or seizures, often for decades.

Of course, there are also many women who are fortunate enough never to experience any problems with their menstrual period, whose period only comes at opportune times, and who enjoy having a period. But even if you're one of these lucky women who values the time of her period as a special, meaningful event, you probably have more in common with the other women than you think. Namely, there's a good chance that *you're basing decisions about your period on inaccurate information.* For example, you might think you always have to have a monthly period to "clean" the womb. (You don't.) Few women know why their period happens or which organs and hormones are involved, much less how to manage their periods. Even worse, many women are basing their decisions on outdated information. For example, can you name a few period-related health benefits? (Hint: There aren't any.) Chances are that, love it or hate it, no matter how you feel about your menstrual period, there are quite a few useful things you can use to improve the quality of your life and health.

The problem is there are no handy, reliable resources available with information about managing your period: only one book that mentions menstrual management was published last year. In contrast, almost fifty dog care books came out. Don't get me wrong, I'm as much a lover of dogs as the next person, as my two spoiled, slightly overweight dogs could attest to. However, information for dog owners shouldn't take precedence over the informational needs of millions of women. Of course, it's not just the scarcity of books that contribute to the problem. A lot of other factors play a role—from questionable menstrual myths, to the medical community, to the media, to the government. Regardless of who's at fault, the results are the same: hardly any information about managing your period is available and most of that information is either obsolete or incorrect. As a result, you and millions of other women are deprived of the opportunity to make informed decisions about your lifestyle and health.

The good news is you can become informed about your period and menstrual management and, in the process, gain a better understanding of how your body works. You can also learn how to take control of your menstrual period and manage it. This will allow you to become an active participant in choosing what is best for you. In consultation with your physician, you'll be able to decide with confidence if you'd like to use period management to control when your period starts and how many periods you have, or if you should do away with your period altogether for a while.

At this time, it's important to make one thing very clear. If you're looking for a book that offers an opinion about how wonderful or how awful it is to have a period, or how taking control of your period will either save or ruin your life, please carry on. The period is simply a body function and menstrual management is one tool at your disposal. How you feel about your period is unique to you. For anyone else to even suggest how you should feel about it is quite presumptuous. Similarly, whether (and if so, exactly how) using menstrual management could be beneficial to you depends on your particular circumstances. If you want a handy menstrual management guide you can rely on in real life, this is the book for you.

Take Control of Your Period provides you with the type of practical information that lets you become an active participant in decisions affecting your lifestyle and your health. After an introduction to the basics of menstrual management, and the nuts and bolts of the monthly cycle, the book shows you, in detail, how period control works. A number of other topics that are helpful in deciding if menstrual management is beneficial to you, like the reason why women have periods, and the difference between the real and the fake period, are also discussed. Last, but not least, the most common period myths are debunked and the future of menstrual management is spotlighted.

There are many things in our lives over which we have little or no control. The monthly menstrual period doesn't have to be one of them. By investing a little of your time in reading this book you can learn everything you need to know about your period and menstrual management. This, in turn, will allow you to take control of your period and make truly informed decisions to improve your life and health.

1

The Elephant in the Room

An Introduction to Menstrual Management

* * *

The year is 1957 and one little pill is about to change our society. The birth control pill, the first pill designed to prevent pregnancy, has just been invented and submitted for regulatory approval to the Federal Drug Administration (FDA). That is, it has been submitted as a pill to be used for the management of period problems, not for birth control. That's right: not only is the concept of menstrual management time-tested, but the use of the Pill for period control also came before its use for pregnancy control.

What Is Menstrual Management?

So, what is menstrual management, and why have you and many other women never even heard about it? In a nutshell, menstrual management is the ability to control your period. Period control allows you to choose:

* How many periods you have, if any at all (whether to have a period)

* How often you have a period (the period frequency)

* When your period starts (the timing of the period)

* More or less, the number of days you menstruate and how much (the duration and amount of flow)

Of course, the degree of control you have with menstrual management is not absolute. (But, then again, what in life is?) In general, it's easier to precisely control whether or not you have a period, and how often, than it is to manage its exact timing, duration, and the amount of flow. For example, let's say you need to skip your period for six months because you have a medical problem, like very painful periods (dysmenorrhea). Using menstrual management allows you to stop having periods for those six months. On the other hand, if you want your period to start exactly on Saturday, February 21, at 11 A.M. because you're scheduled to depart on your spring break exactly two weeks later to the hour, menstrual management gives you an approximate, not absolute degree of control. The good news is by learning about menstrual management and by taking advantage of its various options, you can gain a great deal of control over your period.

When Do You Use Menstrual Management, How Often, and For How Long?

So, menstrual management is the ability to control your period, and the degree of control you have depends on what aspect of the period you want to manage. But when do you use menstrual management, and how often?

The answer to the first part of the question is easy: you use menstrual management whenever you want to or need to. Later in this chapter, we'll discuss in more detail the host of reasons to use period control, but for now we can generalize and divide these reasons into two broad categories:

* Lifestyle—major life events, jobs, vacations, and personal preference

* Health—"minor" period problems, period-related health conditions, various diseases, and before surgery or chemotherapy

Obviously, each woman will have her own reasons for using period management. And, not surprising, those reasons may change throughout her life. For example, in your teens you might use period control for therapeutic reasons, in your twenties and thirties you might use it to deal with lifestyle issues, while in your forties you might use it for a combination of therapeutic and lifestyle reasons. As these reasons change, both the frequency and duration of how you use menstrual management will change as well. (We'll discuss in detail the frequency and duration of the various regimens in chapters 5 and 6.)

What Is Used for Menstrual Management?

At first glance, the idea that it's possible to manage your period might seem odd. That's understandable given that generations of women have viewed their menstrual periods as a grand and inevitable yet mysterious occurrence. That's unfortunate since it's something most of us experience on a regular basis for more than thirty-five years. The truth of the matter is if you understand how the menstrual cycle works, it's easy to understand how menstrual management works, too.

Without going into a lot of detail here (we'll do that in later chapters), your menstrual period is controlled by both nature and nurture:

* Nature—reproduction of the species, body hormones

* Nurture—societal factors, such as whether you live in an agricultural or industrial society, the quality of health care, etc.

In order for you to control your menstrual period, you need to use either hormones or societal factors. Societal factors are an impractical way to manage periods—shifting an agrarian society to an industrial one is quite an undertaking for one person. In contrast, once synthetic (man-made) hormones were invented, it became relatively easy to mimic the nature part. Just as the body controls the start, frequency, and duration of the period by increasing and decreasing the levels of various natural hormones, women can achieve the same results by using various drugs similar to the body's hormones. We'll discuss these natural and societal factors, as well as the menstrual management drugs and how they control the period, in detail later on.

For now, it's important for you to understand one thing: there's nothing mysterious or odd about menstrual management. All you're doing is imitating nature. (For a discussion of what's natural vs. normal when it comes to menstrual periods, see chapter 3.) On a related note, there's another important thing for you to understand. Menstrual management is neither good nor bad. It's simply a tool at your disposal. The same is also true about whether you should use period control, as well as the benefits you might derive from using it. More on this later.

Now that we've covered the basics of menstrual management, let's see who should use period control, what it can do for you, and its advantages and drawbacks.

Who Should Use Menstrual Management?

In general, the reasons for using menstrual management can be grouped into managing lifestyle issues and managing health problems.

Lifestyle reasons for using period control range from simply not liking a monthly period to attempting to integrate in a society that discriminates against menstruating women. Other reasons include leading an active lifestyle, taking part in an upcoming life event, participating in sports or recreational activities, improving school or job performance, and easing the daily life of women with developmental disabilities, for example, women with moderate to severe mental retardation.

Health reasons for using menstrual management include dealing with common period problems—cramps, bloating, breast tenderness, ovulation pain (mittelschmerz), nausea and vomiting, and premenstrual syndrome (PMS)—as well as treating period-related medical conditions and conditions that are worsened by having a period, such as:

* Heavy and painful periods

* Premenstrual syndrome (PMS) and premenstrual dysphoric disorder (PMMD)

* Migraine headaches and seizures

* Endometriosis

* Uterine fibroids

* Adenomyosis (a condition in which tissue normally lining the cavity of the uterus grows inside its muscle wall instead)

* Anemias (iron-deficiency, sickle cell)

* Bleeding disorders and blood diseases (von Willebrand's idiopathic thrombocytopenic purpura [ITP])

* HIV/AIDS and hepatitis B and C

Of course, in real life, the distinction between these two categories isn't always clear-cut and depends on a woman's unique circumstance; your lifestyle issue may be another woman's health problem. For example, a woman with a high pain tolerance might consider painful periods a lifestyle issue because she's able to deal with the inconvenience. However, for another woman, who is more sensitive to pain and who has a very physically demanding job, painful periods are a medical issue.

Many specific groups of women can benefit, for any of these reasons, from menstrual management:

WOMEN WHO DON'T WANT TO HAVE MONTHLY PERIODS

Obviously, one group of women who can greatly benefit from using menstrual management is women who don't want to have monthly periods—either because they simply don't like to or because they live in societies that consider menstruating women "untouchable."

If you think that most women are somehow deeply enamored with their monthly periods and want to bleed every month, think again. In various studies, surveys, and polls, this is what women had to say when asked, "How often do you want to have a period?":

* Eighty-two percent of women want to have their period every three months. (1977 British study)

* Seventy percent of women said they would eliminate the period completely or at least have it less frequently than once a month. (1999 Dutch survey)

* Overall, 44 percent of women would prefer never to have a period, increasing to 59 percent for women aged 40 to 49. (2002 U.S. poll)

* Twenty-nine percent of women do prefer to have a monthly period. (2002 U.S. poll)

In a nutshell, what the studies, surveys, and polls found is that the preferred frequency of bleeding is every three months, closely followed by: never.

WOMEN WHO HAVE AN ACTIVE LIFESTYLE

At the start of Operation Iraqi Freedom, Staff Sergeant Melanie S., a U.S. Marine, baked in 120-degree temperatures, routinely scanned for a tree or shrub that would offer some privacy during a toilet break, twisted into odd shapes to catch foxhole naps, and withstood sand and ever-present insects. As if that wasn't enough, the staff sergeant also had to cope with having her period in a combat zone. When her supply of tampons and pads ran out, she was also faced with constantly scrounging for anything even remotely resembling a suitable replacement. After her return to the States, Melanie said something that summed it up best: "Where was menstrual management when I needed it in Iraq?"

---

* FAST FACT

There are more than 170,000 active-duty servicewomen in the U.S. military, comprising almost 15 percent of the total active force.

Clearly, one group of women who can greatly benefit from using period control is women in the military. But women in the military aren't the only women who lead active lifestyles. Avid surfers, stay-at-home mothers, and women who enjoy active vacations are all good candidates for menstrual management. There are also the millions of women with physically demanding jobs—shift factory workers, scientists working in remote areas, lawyers, airline pilots and flight crew, policewomen, nurses, teachers, performing artists, and mail carriers, to mention just a few.

WOMEN WITH PERIOD-RELATED HEALTH PROBLEMS

Not all women have the luxury of choosing whether to use menstrual management. A large group of women needs to use period control—the millions of women who suffer from period-related health problems.

Most women are all too familiar with the common monthly period problems: cramps, breast tenderness, nausea and vomiting, bloating, and premenstrual syndrome (PMS), to name just a few. Although arguably not life-threatening ailments, any of these so-called minor period problems can, at one time or another, constitute a serious problem.

Of course, many other women also suffer from serious, potentially life-threatening period-related conditions like anemia, debilitatingly painful periods, endometriosis, bleeding disorders, seizures, and uterine fibroids. For these women, menstrual management is essential for good health.

> ✳ **FAST FACT**
> Period-related disorders are the most common gynecological problem in the United States, affecting 2.5 million women aged 18 to 50 years.

TEENAGERS AND PERIMENOPAUSAL WOMEN

Jessica, a very sweet fifteen-year-old, always came to see me with her mother, Mrs. T. Over the years, I noticed a marked change in both. Jessica used to be very outgoing and talkative. She was a good student, loved school, participated in a lot of extracurricular activities, and had a lot of friends. However, she gradually became more withdrawn, dropped out of most school activities, and stopped hanging out with most of her friends. The shift coincided with the start of her monthly periods. At first, Jessica was excited about getting her first period, but her periods were heavy, irregular, and lasted anywhere from seven to ten days each month. She soon became exhausted from trying to keep up with her schoolwork and after-school commitments in between episodes of heavy bleeding. At the same time I was taking care of Jessica I was also treating her mother. Mrs. T., at forty-six years old, led a very active life and had always been in good health. However, Mrs. T. started to experience irregular periods, hot flashes, and prolonged bleeding episodes, and a test revealed decreased bone mass. All these problems had slowed her down considerably, and she was miserable.

Jessica and her mother are the perfect examples of two groups of women—teenagers and perimenopausal women—who can benefit from using menstrual management. Women at both poles of the menstrual age are more likely to experience period-related problems, which makes sense if you think about it. Both groups are in a transition stage—teenagers, from no period to their first period (menarche); perimenopausal women, from years of monthly periods to the last period and menopause. The years just after menarche and those leading up to menopause are the times women are very likely to experience problem periods, like irregular and prolonged periods, heavy bleeding and cramps, hot flushes and acne, to name just a few. For many women, menstrual management can reduce the severity of these symptoms.

NONMENSTRUATING WOMEN

Another group of women who can use menstrual management are women who don't have menstrual periods. Intrigued? Read on. In the United States alone there are more than 10 million women who don't have menstrual periods, despite the fact that they belong to the menstruating-women age group and they're perfectly healthy. What all these women have in common, and the reason they don't have a period, is that they're using a form of hormonal birth control, like the Pill.

When a woman uses the Pill for birth control she stops having menstrual periods for the entire time she takes it. (If she uses the Pill for five years, she doesn't have periods for five years.) This is the way hormonal birth control works, and it's perfectly normal. But although these women no longer have a "real" period, most still experience a "fake period"—a monthly bleeding episode and its attendant problems. (This built-in fake period was originally intended to make the Pill seem more natural.) Unfortunately, the problems that accompany the fake period can be quite real. These problems include pain, cramping, and headaches. Fortunately, by using menstrual management, this group of women can control their fake period–related problems. (More on the difference between the real and the fake period in chapter 4.)

WOMEN WHO AREN'T SEXUALLY ACTIVE

Do you think only women who are sexually active can use menstrual management? If your answer is yes, you might be surprised to learn that this isn't correct. Your level of sexual activity, or lack thereof, has nothing to do with the potential benefits of menstrual management.

You can be a virgin—nuns are a group who can benefit from using period control—and use menstrual management, or you can be a mother of four and use it. The reason is quite simple: one drug can have several uses. Just because hormonal birth control can be used for pregnancy protection doesn't mean there's a sexual activity "requirement" built in in order to use menstrual management.

SEXUALLY ACTIVE WOMEN

Doctor Emily H., a cardiologist, is one of the best physicians I have ever met. A brilliant mind combined with a friendly bedside manner and cheerful disposition makes Dr. H. a favorite with patients and colleagues. When I first met her, she was preparing for her wedding and honeymoon. Although she was excited about getting married, Emily wasn't ready to have children, so she was on the Pill. However, in all the prenuptial excitement, Emily almost forgot her fake period was due to start the day she was scheduled to leave on her honeymoon. She urgently needed a refresher course in menstrual management. Luckily, we talked and the honeymoon disaster was averted. We also covered another of her concerns—using menstrual management and birth control at the same time.

Just like women who aren't sexually active, women who are sexually active are a diverse group. Of course, one additional need many sexually active women have is pregnancy prevention. Which brings an additional concern for these women—how will the method of birth control they use fit in with the menstrual management drugs they plan to use? Since there are eight distinct birth control groups, with more than eighty types of individual methods, this is an important concern. In later chapters we'll go into more detail about using menstrual management and birth control at the same time.

Who Shouldn't Use Menstrual Management?

So far we've discussed who can use menstrual management. Let's now shift gears and see who can't use it. This is simple—there's no reason why most women can't use it. One exception, however, is women with an iron overload disease called hemochromatosis. (See chapter 3.) Also, some women should not use certain period-control methods because they may not respond well to them. Luckily, several choices are available so most women can reduce or eliminate side effects by simply switching to a different type of drug. (We'll go over the various period-control drugs in chapters 5 and 6.)

Outside of these two exceptions, the decision typically comes down to personal choice. Some women enjoy their periods, others welcome their period because they like to take an occasional break from sexual intercourse and it's a convenient time to do so, and other sexually active women like to have a monthly period because it offers additional reassurance that they are not pregnant. For these women, use of short-term menstrual management may be right (such as planning a period-free honeymoon), but extended use is not a good match.

Advantages of Using Menstrual Management

CONVENIENCE, AND EVEN SURVIVAL

If you happen to live in a free society and don't like having monthly periods, menstrual management allows you the convenience to decide whether and how often to have a period—once every few months, twice a year, or once every few years. Of course, for millions of women who live in societies where menstruating women are treated as untouchable, the practice of menstrual management has to do less with women's health than with their sense of personal well-being. The advantage of using period control for these women is that of social integration and acceptance, and, in some cases (see the box for an example of severe conditions), even survival.

Menstrual management is also advantageous for women with developmental disabilities, such as those with moderate to severe mental retardation. Period control helps these women and their caretakers deal with issues like personal hygiene and the spread of blood-borne infections.

IMPROVED JOB PERFORMANCE

Regardless of whether your job is to graduate from college, finish a rush project under budget, or take care of two young children, using menstrual management can improve your productivity and make your job easier.

Menstrual management can even have a beneficial impact on the overall economy. One study found that the costs of period-related disorders to U.S. industry are an estimated 8 percent of the total wage bill and can even impact industrial output.

RELIEF FROM PERIOD- AND FAKE PERIOD–RELATED PROBLEMS

About 85 percent of menstruating women experience some degree of premenstrual or menstrual problems. For up to one-third of women, these problems interfere with daily activities. Moreover, even women who are already using the Pill for birth control experience the same type of problems during the placebo week (the week with hormone-free pills). Using menstrual management helps relieve both period- and fake period–related problems like cramps, bloating, breast tenderness, nausea and vomiting, and premenstrual syndrome (PMS).

> * **FAST FACT**
> Using period control helps relieve placebo-related problems in 74 percent of women using the Pill.

HELP FOR MEDICAL CONDITIONS

Menstrual management benefits women with heavy or painful periods, endometriosis, migraine headaches, anemia, and epilepsy, to name just a few. In addition, using period control before certain scheduled surgical procedures, like a hysteroscopy or endometrial ablation, offers the advantage of decreased complications. Women who have to undergo chemotherapy, such as that required before a bone marrow transplant, may also be able to benefit from menstrual management.

> * **DEFINITIONS**
> During a hysteroscopy, a fiberoptic scope is moved through the vagina into the uterus to view the cavity of the uterus or to perform surgery. During an endometrial ablation, part of the lining of the uterine cavity is removed.

Additional, Method-Specific Advantages

Depending on what menstrual management method and regimen you use, you'll be able to benefit from a number of method-related advantages. For example, if you use the Pill, you will benefit from a decreased risk of cancer, pelvic inflammatory disease (PID), and bone density loss, among other things.

✳ FAST FACT

The combination birth control pill reduces your risk of developing ovarian cancer by 40 percent, developing uterine cancer by 50 percent, and being hospitalized for PID by 60 percent. (We'll discuss in detail all the method-related advantages in chapters 5 and 6.)

✳ DEFINITION

Pelvic inflammatory disease (PID) is an infection of the upper part of a woman's reproductive organs (usually involving the fallopian tubes). PID can cause problems with fertility and abnormal (ectopic) pregnancies, and must be treated with antibiotics as soon as possible.

DECREASED RISK OF TOXIC SHOCK SYNDROME (TSS)

Period-related cases of toxic shock syndrome (TSS) account for 50–70 percent of all cases of TSS in women of reproductive age. Although the risk of TSS is low, if you're a tampon user you have greater than tenfold the risk of developing TSS compared to women who do not use tampons. Obviously, if you use menstrual management and don't have a period at all or less frequently, your need to use tampons is reduced and so is your risk of developing TSS.

BETTER PREGNANCY PROTECTION

For women who are sexually active, one of the potential advantages of menstrual management is better pregnancy protection. For example, women who use the Pill for birth control take a hormone pill for three weeks in a row, followed by a hormone-free (placebo) pill for one week. As any woman who has used the Pill knows, it's relatively easy to miss taking one or more pills. Of course, every time you forget to take a pill, you put yourself at risk for an unwanted pregnancy, especially if the pills missed are the ones just after the placebo week. The reason you're at risk for pregnancy at this time is because, without the Pill, the ovary can quickly release a mature egg. A mature egg plus sperm equals a possible future baby.

The advantage of using menstrual management is that, if you're using the Pill, you take it continuously. So, for example, if you want to bleed only every three months, you take a hormone pill every day, without a placebo break, for three months. (The placebo week comes at the end of the three months.) As a result, the chance that an egg will be released because of a missed pill is greatly reduced. You're better protected against an unintended pregnancy. Of course, a related benefit of the better pregnancy protection is a decreased likelihood of having to have an abortion to terminate an unintended pregnancy.

If you use a continuous menstrual management Pill regimen (the 49-day option), your yearly spending on feminine hygiene products is almost half that of a woman who uses a regular, 28-day birth control regimen: $17.54 per year for the period control regimen compared to $41.45 for the birth control regimen. The trips to the store to purchase these items, the need to prod loved ones to make an emergency run for you, and the chances of accidentally ruining clothes are also reduced when you use menstrual management.

Of course, these advantages have to be balanced with the need to buy extra packs of pills. It all depends on what type of menstrual management you use. For example, one study found that—assuming an average use of eighteen tampons per month—using a trimonthly menstrual management pill regimen (taking a pill continuously for three months) is cost effective if the cost of a pill pack to you is $9.45. (We'll go over the menstrual management regimens in detail in chapters 5 and 6.)

No review of the basics of menstrual management would be complete without addressing its obvious "elephant in the room" characteristic. After all, period control has been around for almost half a century, most women obstetrician/gynecologists use it, for themselves and their patients, yet, despite all this, most women, and quite a few health-care professionals don't know about it. Why is that?

✳ FAST FACT

In the United States there are about 5.38 million pregnancies each year. About half, or 2.65 million, are unintended pregnancies. Of these unintended pregnancies, the majority (1.4 million) end in abortion.

Disadvantages of Using Menstrual Management

As with everything else in life, if something has advantages it also has disadvantages. Here are some of the real and perceived drawbacks of using menstrual management.

SPOTTING

The most common drawback of menstrual management, and a common reason women stop using it, is breakthrough spotting or bleeding. (For a detailed discussion of breakthrough spotting see chapter 4.) The spotting usually occurs when you first start using period control, especially if you've never used a hormonal method before. Your body needs time to adjust to the new regimen. You're most likely to experience spotting during the first three months of use.

One study that looked at the number of spotting days in two groups of women—those using the Pill for menstrual management and those using it for birth control—found that during the first three months of use, women in the first group spotted for six days compared to four days for those in the second group. However, by the end of the one-year study no difference in spotting was found. Fortunately, for the majority of women (72 percent in the afore-mentioned study) the spotting disappears after the first few months of use. In fact, studies have found that, overall, women who use the Pill for menstrual management have fewer spotting days than do women who use it for pregnancy prevention.

DRUG SIDE EFFECTS

When you manage your period you have a choice of using any one of a number of methods that contain synthetic hormones. The Pill is one example. Just like natural hormones, man-made hormones can cause side effects. For example, too much natural estrogen can cause cancer of the uterus. Similarly, in some women, synthetic estrogen has been associated with an increased risk of developing blood clots (deep vein thrombosis [DVT]). Although the risk of experiencing the serious side effects associated with hormonal use is small, if you de-cide to use any of the methods, you should be aware of them.

DELAYED SIGN OF PREGNANCY

If you're sexually active and you rely on your monthly period as a sign that you're not pregnant, obviously not having a period every month is a drawback. Of course, missed periods aren't a great pregnancy diagnosis tool. However, if you're a woman who feels comforted by your monthly period as a sign that you're not pregnant, here are two helpful things to consider: First, a pregnancy is even less likely to occur on the continuous regimen used for menstrual management than it is on the "on/off" regimen used for birth control—less chance of a mature egg being released if you forget to take a pill. Second, if you're using menstrual management and no longer have monthly periods, you can look for other signs of pregnancy, such as nausea, breast tenderness, fatigue, and frequent urination. Of course, it goes without saying that if you suspect that you're pregnant you should take a pregnancy test and check with your physician.

LACK OF MANUFACTURERS' DIRECTIONS

Most brands and methods of birth control don't come with instructions for menstrual management. At the time of this writing, only one pill brand, Seasonale, has been approved by the FDA for menstrual management use. This means this is the only brand that can be used on-label for period control and, as such, it's the only brand specifically packaged with instructions for period control. (Remember, unless a drug's use is an on-label use, the drug manufacturer isn't allowed to directly communicate with you about it.)

The good news is most of the regular (monophasic) combination birth control pill brands can be used for period control. (There are more than ten brands with the exact same formulation as Seasonale.) Not to mention that there are a host of other methods, like the skin patch (Ortho Evra), the vaginal ring (NuvaRing), shots, implants, and hormone-releasing intrauterine devices (IUDs), that can be used to control your period. However, if you use any of these methods, you'll need to get the instructions from your doctor or health-care professional. In chapters 5 and 6, we'll also go over basic instructions for these methods.

> ✳ **DEFINITIONS**
>
> A "monophasic" birth control pill brand is a brand in which each active pill (the hormone-containing pills) has the same amount of hormones. The other types of pill brands are "biphasic" and "triphasic." (For a detailed explanation see chapter 5.)

LACK OF LONG-TERM STUDIES FOR SOME METHODS AND REGIMENS

Various hormonal birth control methods, dosages, and regimens can be used for menstrual management. (We'll discuss in detail the methods, dosages, and regimens used for period control in later chapters.) However, because some of them are relatively new, more long-term studies of their use in menstrual management will be beneficial. For example, two hormonal birth control methods, the skin patch (Ortho Evra) and the vaginal ring (NuvaRing), were developed and approved for pregnancy control and made available relatively recently.

METHOD	FDA APPROVAL/AVAILABILITY
Pill	1960
Vaginal ring (NuvaRing)	2001
Skin patch (Ortho Evra)	2002

Although both the ring and the patch use the same type of hormones as the Pill, delivery route is different—through the vagina and the skin. Both methods could be used off-label for extended use. However, neither is backed by the same kind of studies as the Pill. (More on this in chapter 4.)

NEGATIVE VIEW OF MENSTRUATION

Some people believe that widespread use of menstrual management will result in a negative view of menstruation. I disagree. The menstrual period is a normal body function and menstrual management is simply a tool at your disposal. You use period control when it benefits your lifestyle and/or health, not because periods are "bad" or "evil." Depending on your particular circumstances, using it can be advantageous or disadvantageous for you.

Who Is Not Telling You about Menstrual Management (and Why That Should Concern You)

Physicians have used menstrual management for almost half a century to help their patients manage everything from lifestyle to life-threatening medical conditions. And yet, period control has only recently come out of the closet. Why? Well, the short, diplomatic answer is: for any number of reasons.

HEALTH-CARE PROFESSIONALS

The average doctor's visit in the United States lasts about fifteen minutes—too short a time for lengthy explanations or a lot of patient questions. Additionally, health-care professionals are under increasing pressure to act less like healers and more like potential defendants. As a result, many are reluctant to suggest off-label uses of drugs to their patients. (For the meaning of "off-label" use, see

> ✳ **FAST FACT**
> In a survey of nurses and physicians, 43 percent of participants said they don't prescribe drugs for menstrual management because patients don't ask for them; 4 percent don't prescribe them because of the extra counseling time involved; and 4 percent mentioned legal worries ("off-label" use) as their reason for not prescribing.

the box below.) Moreover, within the medical profession, the doctors who have a thorough understanding of menstrual management and who use it routinely for their patients or for themselves are a relative minority.

THE GOVERNMENT AND PHARMACEUTICAL COMPANIES

Until recently, using hormonal birth control (commonly used menstrual management drugs) for period control was an "off-label" use. On September 5, 2003, the FDA approved Seasonale (Barr Laboratories), the first brand of pill specifically packaged for menstrual management.

❊ DEFINITIONS

What do "off-label" and "on-label" mean? Here's an example illustrating the definitions. The antidepressant drug Zoloft is FDA-approved for treating depression. This is an "on-label" use. While using it, physicians notice that it's also very effective at treating premature ejaculation and start using it for that as well. This is an "off-label" use. Only drugs that are already FDA-approved can be used off-label.

How does the off-label designation contribute to the problem? It keeps you out of the loop by law. Pharmaceutical companies are not allowed to distribute information about off-label uses to the public, and many times they don't volunteer the information to health-care professionals, either.

Moreover, for the FDA to approve the change from an off-label use of a drug to an on-label one, the drug manufacturer has to conduct additional studies that show the drug is successful in treating whatever off-label condition it's used for. Additional studies mean untold additional millions of dollars for the manufacturer, and the approval process can take years. However, because the drug is already FDA-approved, physicians are already using it, legally, off-label (they can even be sued for malpractice if they don't). As a result, the drug manufacturer often has little incentive to invest in changing the drug's designation.

Until recently, this unfortunate combination of factors kept many women uninformed about menstrual management. (After all, it's impossible to ask your doctor about the benefits of a technique you don't know exists.) The good news is twofold: both the government and the drug manufacturers are stepping up to the plate and making an effort to correct this problem. The FDA has instituted new application procedures to expedite drug approval; and drug manufacturers, such as Barr Laboratories, Johnson & Johnson, and Schering AG, are all developing new menstrual management drugs.

THE MEDIA AND SOCIETY

"Brace yourself. This is a commercial about your period!" A variant of this advisory comes at the start of almost every TV commercial for feminine hygiene products. Why exactly do you need to "brace yourself"? Commercials about dental plaque, bladder leakage, gas, acid reflux, and impotence offer no such advance warning. The message here seems to be that the menstrual period is more disgusting than any other known bodily function (and a few dysfunctions, as well).

Granted, there are people who would prefer there never be any public discussion of bodily functions. I also realize that, unlike most people, I have a high level of tolerance for these matters because I'm an obstetrician/gynecologist. However, the question remains, why is the menstrual period the ugly stepsister of bodily functions? A likely answer is that old views die hard. Before the menstrual period was fully understood, it was viewed as a mysterious yet regular event that didn't kill the women who experienced it, while any bleeding in men most likely resulted in their death. The end result was a certain degree of squeamishness toward periods. Until this mindset changes, the lack of informative period-related stories in the media and in society will continue to contribute to keeping women in the dark about menstrual management.

The good news is that there are signs of change. About the time that Seasonale was approved by the FDA, all the major newspapers and wire services, and even TV stations, dedicated at least a story to the subject of menstrual management. The stories still contained some mistakes, but at least none carried an advisory at the beginning of the story.

Just because a number of factors have contributed to lack of information about menstrual management, it doesn't mean we have to accept being in the dark about this important subject. Menstrual management has enormous potential to positively affect both your health and your lifestyle. And this is why it makes sense to invest a little bit of time learning about whether the technique is right for you either now or in the future.

The menstrual period is a major part of every woman's life. Surprisingly, women routinely arm themselves with a great deal more information about things that feature far less prominently in their lives, such as comparison-shopping for household appliances. Something that will be with you for over a third of your life deserves no less consideration.

Last, but not least, *being informed* about menstrual management allows you to *make an informed decision* about whether you should use period control. Already, in addition to Seasonale, researchers at a number of institutions are working on the next generation of period control drugs. The more you know about menstrual management the more input you have. There's no reason why you can't or shouldn't become an active participant, in consultation with your physician, in decisions that affect your lifestyle and health, as well as those of your loved ones.

Chapter One Bibliography

[FDA's] Approval of the Oral Contraceptive by Suzanne White Junoa. FDLI Update. 1998;4:10.

Who Should Use Menstrual Management

Burkman RT, Miller L. Extended and continuous use of hormonal contraceptives. *Dialogues Contracept.* Winter 2004;8(4):1–8.

Kaunitz AM, Sulak, PJ. Amenorrhea and hormonal contraception. *Dialogues Contracept.* Spring 2002;7(4):1–3.

Kaunitz AM, Westhoff C, Coddington III CC, *et al.* Regulating menstruation: impact on lifestyle and medical conditions. *Female Patient.* 2002 Apr;27 (4Suppl):8–11.

Hillard PJA. When should you induce amenorrhea? *Contemp Ob/Gyn.* 2003 Jun;48(6):60–72.

Fraser IS, Kovacs GT. The efficacy of non-contraceptive uses for hormonal contraceptives. *MJA* 2003;178(12):621–3.

Freeman EW. Evaluation of a unique oral contraceptive (Yasmin) in the management of premenstrual dysphoric disorder. *Eur J Contracept Reprod Health Care.* 2002 Dec;7 Suppl 3:27–34; discussion 42–3.

WOMEN WHO DON'T WANT TO HAVE A MONTHLY PERIOD

Loudon NB, Foxwell M, Potts DM, *et al.* Acceptability of an oral contraceptive that reduces the frequency of menstruation: the tri-cycle pill regimen. *Br Med J.* 1977;2:487–90.

den Tonkelar I, Oddens BJ. Preferred frequency and characteristics of menstrual bleeding in relation to reproductive status, oral contraceptive use, and hormone replacement therapy use. *Contraception.* 1999;59: 357–62.

Association of Reproductive Health Professionals. Extended regimen oral contraceptives. Harris Poll. June 14–17, 2002.

WOMEN WHO HAVE AN ACTIVE LIFESTYLE

28th Annual Department of Defense Report. Population representation in the military services. Active component enlisted force: Gender. 3–7.

Schneider MB, Fisher M, Friedman SB, *et al.* Menstrual and premenstrual issues in female military cadets: a unique population with significant concerns. *J Pediatr Adolesc Gynecol.* 1999;12:195–201.

WOMEN WITH PERIOD-RELATED HEALTH PROBLEMS

Hatcher RA, Guillebaud MA. The pill: combined oral contraceptives. In: Hatcher RA, Trussell J, Stewart F, *et al.*, eds. *Contraceptive Technology*. New York: Ardent Media; 1998: 405–66.

Kjerulff KH, Erickson BA, Langenberg PW. Chronic gynecological conditions reported by US women: findings from the National Health Interview Survey, 1984 to 1992. *Am J Public Health*. 1996;86:195–9.

Piccinino LJ, Mosher WD. Trends in contraceptive use in the United States: 1982–1995. *Fam Plann Perspect*. 1998;30(1):4–10 and 46.

TEENAGERS AND PERIMENOPAUSAL WOMEN

Kaunitz AM. Oral contraceptive use in perimenopause. *Am J Obstet Gynecol*. 2001;185(2Suppl) 32–7.

Kaunitz AM, Westhoff C, Coddington III CC, *et al*, 2002, op cit.

Sulak PJ. Creative use of oral contraceptives: perimenopause, menstrual disorders, premenstrual syndrome, and extended regimens. In: *Understanding Contraceptive Choice: The Patient's Perspective*. November 2003:10–18.

NONMENSTRUATING WOMEN

Piccinino LJ, Mosher WD, 1998, op. cit.

Sulak PJ, Scow RD, Preece C, *et al.* Hormone withdrawal symptoms in oral contraceptive users. *Obstet Gynecol*. 2000 Feb;95(2):261–6.

Sulak PJ, Cressman BE, Waldrop E, *et al.* Extending the duration of active oral contraceptive pills to manage hormone withdrawal symptoms. *Obstet Gynecol*. 1997 Feb;89(2):179–83.

WOMEN WHO AREN'T SEXUALLY ACTIVE

Xu WH, Xiang YB, Ruan ZX, *et al.* Menstrual and reproductive factors and endometrial cancer risk: results from a population-based case-control study in urban Shanghai. *Int J Cancer*. 2004 Feb;108(4): 613–9.

WHO SHOULDN'T USE MENSTRUAL MANAGEMENT

(See chapters 3, 5, and 6.)

CONVENIENCE AND EVEN SURVIVAL

Chhaupadi system: Age Old Superstition by Sanjaya Dhakal. Nepal News.com. Spotlight Vol 23, No 12, Sept 12–18 2003. http://www.nepalnews.com.np/contents/englishweekly/spotlight/2003/sep/sep12/national3.htm. Accessed June 4, 2004.

Kaunitz AM, Westhoff C, Coddington III CC, *et al*, 2000, op. cit.

Hillard PJA, 2003, op. cit.

IMPROVED JOB PERFORMANCE

Thomas SL, Ellertson C. Nuisance or natural and healthy: should monthly menstruation be optional for women? *Lancet*. 2000 Mar;355(9207): 922–4.

RELIEF FROM PERIOD- AND FAKE PERIOD–RELATED PROBLEMS

Kraemer GR, Kraemer RR. Premenstrual syndrome: diagnosis and treatment. *Women's Health*. 1998;7:893–907.

Sulak PJ. Should your patient be on extended-use OCs? *Contemp Ob/Gyn*. 2003 Sept;48(9):34–46.

Sulak PJ, Scow RD, Preece C, *et al*, 2000, op. cit.

Sulak PJ, Cressman BE, Waldrop E, *et al*, 1997, op. cit.

HELP FOR MEDICAL CONDITIONS

(See *Who Should Use Menstrual Management* and chapters 5 and 6.)

Sulak PJ, 2003, op. cit.

Additional, Method-Specific Advantages

Burkman RT, Collins JA, Shulman LP, *et al*. Current perspectives on oral contraceptive use. *Am J Obstet Gynecol*. 2001 Aug;185(2 Suppl):S4–12.

Burkman RT, Kaunitz AM, Shulman LP, *et al*. Oral contraceptives and noncontraceptive benefits: summary and application of data. *Intl J Fertil*. 2000;45:134.

Dayal M, Barnhart KT. Noncontraceptive benefits and therapeutic uses of the oral contraceptive pill. *Semin Repro Med*. 2001;19(4):295–303.

Cunningham GF, Gant NF, Leveno KJ, *et al*, eds. *Williams Obstetrics*, 21st ed. New York, NY: McGraw-Hill; 2001:1525–6.

(See chapters 5 and 6.)

DECREASE RISK OF TOXIC SHOCK SYNDROME (TSS)

Omar HA, Aggarwal S, Perkins KC. Tampon use in young women. *J Pediatr Adolesc Gynecol*. 1998 Aug;11(3):143–6.

Reingold AL. Toxic shock syndrome: an update. *Am J Obstet Gynecol*. 1991 Oct;165(4 Pt 2):1236–9.

Stallones RA. A review of the epidemiologic studies of toxic shock syndrome. *Ann Intern Med*. 1982 Jun;96(6 Pt 2):917–20.

Lanes SF, Poole C, Dreyer NA, *et al*. Toxic shock syndrome, contraceptive methods, and vaginitis. *Am J Obstet Gynecol*. 1986 May;154(5): 989–91.

BETTER PREGNANCY PROTECTION

Henshaw SK. Unintended pregnancy in the United States. *Fam Plann Perspect*. 1998;30(1):24–9 and 46.

SAVINGS ON FEMININE HYGIENE PRODUCTS

Miller L, Notter KM. Menstrual reduction with extended use of combination oral contraceptive pills: randomized controlled trial. *Obstet Gynecol*. 2001 Nov;98(5 Pt 1):771–8.

Schwartz JL, Creinin MD, Pymar HC. The trimonthly combination oral contraceptive regimen: is it cost effective? *Contraception*. 1999 Nov; 60(5):263–7.

SPOTTING

Miller L, Hughes JP. Continuous combination oral contraceptive pills to eliminate withdrawal bleeding: a randomized trial. *Obstet Gynecol*. 2003;101:653–61.

DRUG SIDE EFFECTS

(See chapters 4, 5, and 6.)

Burkman RT, Collins JA, Shulman LP, *et al*, 2001 op. cit.

DELAYED SIGN OF PREGNANCY

Cunningham GF, Gant NF, Leveno KJ, *et al*, eds. *Williams Obstetrics*, 21st ed. New York, NY: McGraw-Hill; 2001:23–9.

LACK OF MANUFACTURERS' DIRECTIONS

FDA Approves Seasonale Oral Contraceptive. FDA Talk Paper T03-65 September 5, 2003.

(See chapters 5 and 6 and Appendix A.)

LACK OF LONG-TERM STUDIES FOR SOME METHODS AND REGIMENS

(See chapters 4 and 5.)

FDA Approves First Hormonal Vaginal Contraceptive Ring. FDA Talk Paper T01-46 October 3, 2001.

FDA Approves First Hormonal Contraceptive Skin Patch. FDA Talk Paper T01-58 November 20, 2001.

United States availability of Ortho Evra, N. Naya, personal communication.

NEGATIVE VIEW OF MENSTRUATION

Review essay by Kathleen O'Grady. http://www.mum.org/ismenob.htm. Accessed May 16, 2004.

USE OF PERIOD CONTROL BY WOMEN OBSTETRICIAN/GYNECOLOGISTS

American College of Obstetricians and Gynecologists. Survey of women obstetrician/gynecologists. Gallup Poll. September 2003.

HEALTHCARE PROFESSIONALS

Bensing JM, Roter DL, Hulsman RL. Communication patterns of primary care physicians in the United States and the Netherlands. *J Gen Intern Med*. 2003 May;18(5):335–42.

Blumenthal D, Causino N, Chang YC, *et al*. The duration of ambulatory visits to physicians. *J Fam Pract*. 1999 Apr;48(4):264–71.

Gilchrist VJ, Stange KC, Flocke SA, *et al*. A comparison of the National Ambulatory Medical Care Survey (NAMCS) measurement approach with direct observation of outpatient visits. *Med Care*. 2004 Mar;42 (3):276–80.

Gross DA, Zyzanski SJ, Borawski EA, *et al*. Patient satisfaction with time spent with their physician. *J Fam Pract*. 1998 Aug; 47(2):133–7.

Association of Reproductive Health Professionals and National Association of Nurse Practitioners in Women's Health. Annual meeting registrant survey. August–September 2002.

Stone KJ, Viera AJ, Parman CL. Off-label applications for SSRIs. *Am Fam Physician* 2003;68(3);498–504.

Palumbo FB, Mullins CD. The development of direct-to-consumer prescription drug advertising regulation. *Food Drug Law J.* 2002;57(3):423–44.

Jagger SF. Prescription drugs: implications of drug labeling and off-label use. Statement before the Subcommittee on Human Resources and Intergovernmental Relations, Committee on Government Reform and Oversight, U.S. House of Representatives. Washington, D.C.: General Accounting Office, 1996. (GAO/T-HEHS-96-212)

DiMasi JA, Hansen RW, Grabowski HG. The price of innovation: new estimates of drug development costs. *J Health Econ.* 2003 Mar;22(2): 151–85.

DiMasi JA, Kaitin KI, Fernandez-Carol C, *et al.* New indications for already-approved drugs: an analysis of regulatory review times. *J Clin Pharmacol.* 1991 Mar;31(3):205–15.

Use of approved drugs for unlabeled indications. FDA Drug Bill 1982; 12(1):4–5. United States Food and Drug Admin., Washington, D.C.

U.S. Food and Drug Administration IRB Information Sheets. Guidance for Institutional Review Boards and Clinical Investigators 1998 Update. "Off-Label" and Investigational Use of Marketed Drugs, Biologics, and Medical Devices. United States Food and Drug Admin., Washington, D.C.

Statement by William B. Schultz, Deputy Commissioner for Policy, FDA, before the Committee on Labor and Human Resources, United States Senate, February 22, 1996. http://www.gao.gov/. Accessed June 6, 2004. (GAO/T-HEHS-96-212)

Cranston JW, Williams MA, Nielsen NH, Bezman RJ, for the Council on Scientific Affairs. Unlabeled indications of Food and Drug Administration-approved drugs. *Drug Inf J.* 1998;32:1049–61.

Nightingale SL. Off-label use of prescription drugs. *Am Fam Physician.* 2003;68 (3):425–7.

Serradell J, Galle B. Prescribing for unlabeled indications. *HMO Pract.* 1993 Mar;7(1):44–7.

Merrill RA. Modernizing the FDA: an incremental revolution. *Health Aff* (Millwood). 1999 Mar–Apr;18(2):96–111.

Kaitin KI, Cairns C. The new drug approvals of 1999, 2000, and 2001: drug development trends a decade after passage of the prescription drug user fee act of 1992. *Drug Inf J* 2003;37(4):357–72.

Barr Laboratories. Selected Proprietary Products in Development. http://www.barrlabs.com/pages/proprietcon.htm. Accessed May 16, 2004.

Freedom from the Menstrual Cycle? Barr Labs is testing a new contraceptive pill that could all but banish monthly bleeding and open new lifestyle options for women by Amy Tsao. Business Week Online, May 23, 2002. http://www.businessweek.com/technology/content/may2002/tc20020523_4148.htm. Accessed May 16, 2004.

Philip Smits, MD. Schering R&D Day 2003. Berlin, 26 June 2003.

THE MEDIA AND SOCIETY

New Pill Fuels Debate Over Benefits of Fewer Periods by Tina Kelley. *The New York Times*, October 14, 2003; Late Edition—Final, Section F, Page 5, Column 2.

FDA Approves New Birth Control Pill by Robe Stein. *The Washington Post Saturday*, September 6, 2003; Page A07.

New Pill Stops Women's Periods. CBS/AP 2003. (WCBS News radio 880. Sep 5, 2003 9:57 pm US/Eastern.)

NO FLOW. The FDA just approved a new birth control pill that will allow women to have periods only four times a year—just as nature intended by Audrey Van Buskirk. theStranger.com. Vol 13 No. 1, Sep 18–Sep 24 2003. http://www.thestranger.com/2003-09-18/feature.html. Accessed May 16, 2004.

From Top to Bottom

The Nuts and Bolts of Your Period and Menstrual Cycle

* * *

Your best friend tells you she's been using menstrual management for a while and that not having a period every month is the greatest thing since sliced bread. But just the other day you read somewhere that it's unnatural for women not to have a monthly period, and the "expert" warned readers that period control can cause big problems. You don't know who to believe.

You need information. You need to understand the "mechanics" of the menstrual period and monthly cycle. Once you do, you'll be able to make an educated decision, in consultation with your physician, about whether menstrual management is right for you. This chapter covers the "nuts and bolts"—the body organs and hormones—involved with your menstrual period and monthly cycle.

When it comes to your menstrual period, the uterus or womb is where all the action is. However, you might be surprised to find out that other organs, from your brain to your vagina, also play a role. Four main body organs are involved with the period:

* *The brain.* The brain has a major connection with your menstrual period—this is where the main chemicals that regulate the period are made. These chemicals are hormones. Hormones control many body functions. During your cycle, the areas of the brain that secrete hormones include the hypothalamus (which produces gonadotropin-releasing hormone, GnRH) and the anterior pituitary (which produces follicle-stimulating hormone, FSH; and luteinizing hormone, LH).

* *The ovaries.* You have two ovaries. They are walnut-shaped organs, one on each side of the upper part of the uterus. Your ovaries make "worker hormones," estrogen and progesterone, as well as the hormone testosterone. The ovaries are also responsible for releasing eggs (*ova*).

* *The uterus.* The uterus, or womb, is a thick-walled, muscular organ, the size of a small, hollow, upside-down pear. It is located deep inside your pelvis. For most women, hormones cause part of the tissue that lines the uterine cavity to shed in the form of menstrual blood once a month (menses, menstruation).

> *** FAST FACT**
> The nonpregnant uterus is about the size of a small closed fist and weighs 1.8 ounces (50 grams). A uterus with a full-term pregnancy is about the size of a large watermelon and weighs 2.4 pounds (1.100 grams).

* *The vagina.* This muscular, tubelike organ connects the uterus to the exterior of a woman's body. In other words, it provides a passageway for the menstrual blood from the uterus to the outside.

The brain is in charge of everything. The ovaries and the uterus are part of the woman's upper genital tract, while the vagina is part of the lower genital tract.

> ✳ **FAST FACT**
>
> A number of birth control methods act at the level of the woman's upper genital tract:
>
> - Hormonal methods affect the ovaries and the uterus.
> - Sterilization ("tying your tubes") involves the fallopian tubes.
> - Intrauterine devices (IUDs) work inside the cavity of the uterus.
> - Barrier methods typically are placed near or on the cervix.
>
> Other methods act on the lower genital tract:
>
> - Some barrier methods are placed in the vagina.
> - Spermicides are also used in the vagina.

A Woman's Genital Tract

Here is a more detailed description of a woman's genital tract, a few of the problems women may encounter, and how menstrual management can help.

Upper Female Genital Tract

The ovaries and uterus (which includes the fallopian tubes and cervix) are part of the upper female genital tract. Except for the cervix, which is partly within the vagina, these organs are located deep within the pelvic cavity.

OVARIES

The ovaries are positioned behind and below the fallopian (uterine) tubes. They release eggs as well as steroid hormones. Usually, one egg is released each month. Eggs are released from an ovarian folli-

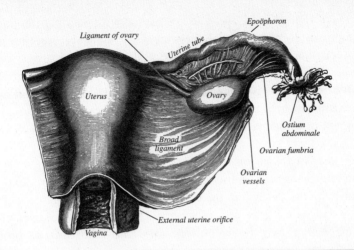

Figure 1 The upper female genital track.
Gray's Anatomy, 1918 Edition

Labels on figure: Ligament of ovary, Uterine tube, Epoöphoron, Uterus, Ovary, Ostium abdominale, Broad ligament, Ovarian fumbria, Ovarian vessels, External uterine orifice, Vagina

cle, the place where the egg matures during the monthly cycle. Think of the follicle as a little egg nest.

CORPUS LUTEUM (YELLOW BODY)

The copus luteum (CL) is not a stand-alone organ; it's an important part of the ovary. Basically, the CL is what's left after the ovarian follicle ruptures and releases the egg. The CL's main function is to release the hormone progesterone. If there's a pregnancy, the CL provides the required progesterone until the placenta (afterbirth) takes over progesterone production. If there's no pregnancy, the CL shrivels up and is called corpus albicans (white body), which is reabsorbed by the body.

Here are a few common ovarian problems women encounter:

Ovarian cysts

When hormone levels fluctuate, a cyst can form in the ovary (functional cyst). Ovarian cysts are most common in women 15 to 44 years old. One study found that 4 percent of menstruating women have cysts larger than 30 millimeters in diameter. Breast cancer patients of reproductive age who are treated with the drug tamoxifen are at greater risk. Although these cysts are not cancerous, they tend to recur and can grow quite large and rupture, causing a lot of pain. These cysts usually resolve on their own; however, when they don't they can require medical intervention. Using menstrual management can help because using the Pill protects against the development of these cysts.

Noncancerous ovarian tumors

Sometimes various tumors, like adenomas, teratomas, and endometriomas, develop in the ovary. Although they're not cancerous, they can cause pain and infertility. Using the Pill for menstrual management may be helpful because the Pill tends to protect against benign ovarian tumors. One study found that in women using the Pill, the risk of these ovarian tumors was reduced by about 20 percent. The risk reduction was greatest for women who had endometrosis-related lesions and for women who had used the Pill for more than twenty-four months. (More about endometriosis when we discuss the uterus.)

Polycystic ovarian syndrome (PCOS)

Polycystic ovarian syndrome (PCOS) is the most common endocrine ("glandular") disorder in women of reproductive age. It affects approximately 4 percent of women. Women with PCOS suffer from irregular bleeding, hirsutism (excessive hair growth in a male pattern), and infertility. Also, women with PCOS are more likely to develop several potentially serious conditions, like diabetes and heart disease. Menstrual management can help because the Pill is one of the treatments for this condition. (Other treatments include diet and exercise, spironolactone ["water pill"], and ovulation induction for infertility.)

UTERUS

The uterus is a hollow, thick-walled, muscular organ deep in the pelvic cavity. (As mentioned earlier, imagine the uterus as a small, hollow pear turned upside down.) Looking at the outside of the uterus, the top—the rounded bottom of the pear—is called the fundus. The lower portion—the neck—is called the cervix. The body, or corpus, lies between the fundus and the cervix. Connected to both sides of the body's upper part are the fallopian tubes (oviducts); the lower part of the uterus (the cervix) connects with the vagina via the uterine opening.

On the inside, the uterus is hollow, and it has very thick, muscular walls. The inner lining is called the endometrium. The uterus has three openings—two on either side of the top area of the body and one in the middle of the neck. The two top openings connect to the fallopian tubes. The bottom opening is the cervical opening, or ostium. The uterus communicates with the vagina through this cervical opening. Menstrual blood flows out of the body through the cervical opening.

The main functions of the uterus are to provide a place for a fertilized egg (an egg that has already united with sperm) to grow and to help push out the fetus during labor. The uterus also plays a role in sexual orgasm—quick, rhythmic contractions of the uterus occur during orgasm. Unfortunately, women can also run into several uterine health problems. The following are a few.

Fibroids

The wall of the uterus is made up of several tissue layers. Most of the thickness is taken up by muscle tissue called myometrium. (In Greek, *myo* means muscle and *metrium* means uterus.) Sometimes this layer starts to grow in knots instead of orderly sheets. These knots are commonly known as fibroids. The majority of fibroids are noncancerous, but some can grow very large and cause pain, infertility, repeated miscarriages, and excessive period bleeding. Fibroids are also a leading reason for surgery to remove the uterus (hysterectomy) in women of childbearing age.

Menstrual management can help women with fibroids by reducing the heavy and/or prolonged bleeding (menorrhagia) they experience. The role of the Pill (a commonly used menstrual management drug) in lowering a woman's risk of fibroids isn't clear—one study found a 31 percent risk reduction in women who had used the Pill for ten years. What is clear is that overall, if you have fibroids, using the Pill doesn't increase their size. This is an important point to remember because there are health professionals who think a history of fibroids is a contraindication to using the Pill. It isn't.

> ✳ **DEFINITION**
>
> The medical name for fibroids is leiomyomas; some other names you might hear used are myomas, fibromyomas, fibroleiomyomas, or fibromas.

Endometriosis

Another important part of the uterine wall is the tissue that lines the cavity of the uterus. This tissue is called the endometrium (*endo* means inside; *metrium* means uterus). It has several layers (the basalis and the functionalis). Each month, under the influence of hormones, part of this tissue (the functionalis) builds up, breaks down, and is eliminated from the body as the menstrual flow. However, sometimes not everything goes according to plan.

Sometimes this tissue grows outside the uterus—on the ovaries, inside the pelvis, on the urinary bladder, in the lungs, or in old surgery scars. This out-of-place tissue (endometriosis) acts as if it were still inside the uterus—it builds up, breaks down, and sheds every month. This poses a problem—the blood and dead tissue have no way to get out of the body; this internal bleeding can cause inflammation, chronic pelvic pain, infertility, and the formation of blood-filled cysts (endometriomas).

> ✳ **FAST FACT**
>
> One theory about the origin of endometriosis is the "retrograde flow" theory. It basically says that instead of flowing out through the lower part of the uterus, some of the menstrual blood reverses direction and flows out of the uterus through the fallopian tubes onto the ovaries or into the pelvic cavity.

In women with endometriosis, the hormonal changes, especially those around the time of the period, can worsen the pelvic pain associated with the disorder. Menstrual management helps by relieving and treating endometriosis problems.

> ✳ **FAST FACT**
>
> Pain is the most common symptom of endometriosis, and nearly 90 percent of women with chronic pelvic pain have endometriosis. As many as 50 percent of infertile women have endometriosis. About one-third of women with endometriosis do not experience symptoms.

FALLOPIAN TUBES (UTERINE TUBES OR OVIDUCTS)

The two fallopian tubes, two hollow tubes one on each side of the uterus, are part of the uterus. One end of each tube connects to the uterus, and the other end has fronds and floats free near the ovary. Each tube is about 10 centimeters long (the size of a bean pod). Fertilization (the union of the egg and sperm) is believed to occur in the outer third of the tube. The main function of a fallopian tube is to transport an egg from an ovary to the uterus, sperm from the uterine cavity into the tube, and the fertilized egg to the uterus.

Ectopic pregnancy

Sometimes a fertilized egg sticks to a surface outside of the uterine cavity and begins to develop. This is called an ectopic pregnancy. The fallopian tubes are one of the most common locations for an ectopic pregnancy. Other sites are the ovary, the abdominal cavity, and the intestines.

Ectopic pregnancies can be life-threatening and require immediate medical attention—they have to be terminated. Depending on the type of ectopic, the treatment can be medical (using drugs) or surgical (either laparoscopic or traditional surgery). Some of the methods used for menstrual management, like the Pill, lower a woman's risk of an ectopic pregnancy.

Pelvic Inflammatory Disease

Pelvic inflammatory disease (PID) is an infection that most commonly involves the fallopian tubes. Untreated sexually transmitted infections (STIs),* like *chlamydia* and *gonorrhea*, often cause PID. Abnormal vaginal discharge, pain and/or tenderness in the lower abdomen and pelvic area—especially during intercourse—and fever and/or chills are symptoms of PID. Unfortunately, some women don't experience any symptoms and don't know they've been infected. This is dangerous because PID can scar fallopian tubes; this, in turn, increases the risk of infertility and ectopic pregnancy.

PID is treated with antibiotics, and the treatment must be started as soon as possible. Of course, your sexual partner must also be tested for STIs and, if found to be infected, treated. If the PID is

---

*The terms sexually transmitted disease (STD) and sexually transmitted infection (STI) are often used interchangeably. In this book we'll use STI.

severe enough (acute PID), hospitalization and intravenous (IV) antibiotics are needed. Acute PID is a medical emergency and about 200,000 women are hospitalized every year with this condition. Some methods used for menstrual management can help by lowering your risk of PID-related hospitalization. (See chapter 5.)

CERVIX

The cervix is the lower part of the uterus and the point of contact between the vagina and the uterus. The cervix provides a passageway for sperm (from the vagina to the uterine cavity), and for menstrual blood and babies (from the uterus to the vagina). One way to think of the cervix is as gateway to the uterus. Some menstrual management methods protect the uterus from infections by "closing" the cervical gate.

✳ FAST FACT

One way hormonal birth control, like the Pill, protects the uterus from infection is by causing the cervical mucus to thicken. In essence, the mucus forms a cervical plug that blocks the entry of infectious agents into the uterus.

Although using the Pill and other hormonal birth control methods decreases the infection rate of some genital infections, if you're sexually active, these methods shouldn't be used as protection against sexually transmitted infections (STIs). A barrier method, like the condom, remains the best available option.

Lower Female Genital Tract

Menstrual management isn't directed at managing lower genital tract problems. However, you might find a brief, practical review of this tract useful.

The organs of the lower female genital tract—the vagina, mons pubis, labia majora and labia minora, and the clitoris—are close to the body surface and partly exposed to the outside.

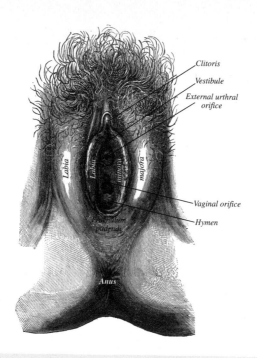

Figure 2 External genital organs of female.
The labia minora have been drawn apart.
Gray's Anatomy, 1918 Edition

VAGINA

The vagina is a muscular, tubelike organ located behind the bladder and in front of the rectum. Its length varies considerably—usually the upper (anterior) wall is 6 to 8 centimeters, and the lower (posterior) wall is 7 to 10 centimeters. The vagina is the passageway from the uterus to the outside world. The vagina also serves as a repository for sperm and plays a role in sexual stimulation, arousal, and orgasm.

The hymen is a thin fold of mucous membrane with a small opening in the middle, which surrounds the vaginal opening. In virgins, menstrual blood passes through the opening in the hymen, which is also flexible enough to allow the passage of menstrual tampons (preferably small or medium ones). If you're unsure how to properly insert a tampon, don't hesitate to ask your health-care professional for help.

The first time a woman has sexual intercourse, small tears can occur in the hymen. The tearing can (but doesn't always) cause a little bit of bleeding. Not surprisingly, this may cause some initial discomfort, but the tears heal by themselves. Because the shape of the hymen varies, its appearance doesn't establish virginity.

The Bartholin glands are two small structures that open just outside the vaginal entrance. These glands produce a small amount of fluid that helps protect the tissue around the vagina and provides lubrication during sexual intercourse. The vaginal bulb is a mass of erectile tissue located deep on either side of the vaginal opening. During intercourse, the bulb fills with blood.

Bartholin gland abscess
The Bartholin glands may occasionally become infected and cause a Bartholin gland abscess. They tend to be uncomfortable and painful, and you need to consult your physician for treatment.

MONS PUBIS
The mons pubis is the external mound of a woman's genitals formed by a collection of fatty tissue right beneath the skin. It becomes covered with hair at the time of puberty.

LABIA MAJORA (BIG LIPS)
The labia majora are the two larger folds of skin that extend downward and backward from the mons pubis. Each lip (labium) has two surfaces: an outer one, pigmented and covered with hairs in adults; and an inner, smooth one. The lips (labia) unite at their upper and lower ends. The space between the place where the labia meet and the anus is called the perineum. The labia majora correspond to the scrotum (testicular sac) in men.

LABIA MINORA (SMALL LIPS)
The labia minora are two small skin folds that extend from the clitoris downward on either side of the vaginal opening. They end be-

tween the vaginal orifice and the labia majora. At its upper end, each small lip (labium minus) divides, and part of the division forms a fold (preputium clitoridis) that overhangs the tip of the clitoris (glans clitoridis).

CLITORIS

The clitoris is an erectile structure under the upper junction of the labia majora and partially hidden between the upper ends of the labia minora. It consists of two corpora cavernosa, composed of erectile tissue. The tip of the clitoris, called the glans clitoridis, is a small rounded nodule that is highly sensitive. The clitoris corresponds to the penis in men.

The labia majora and minora and the clitoris play a role in sexual arousal, stimulation, and orgasm.

EXTERNAL URETHRAL ORIFICE

The urethra, part of the genitourinary tract, is a thin tube that allows the passage of urine. It is connected to the bladder at one end and to the outside via the external urethral opening at the other. The external opening looks like a small cleft with slightly raised margins. It is behind the glans clitoridis and in front of the vaginal opening.

Your Sex Hormones

Virtually every single body function, from thinking to going to the bathroom, is controlled by hormones. Hormones can be either naturally occurring substances (like the ones made by your body) or synthetic compounds (like the ones found in birth control pills). Natural hormones regulate your menstrual period. When you manage your period, you use drugs that contain man-made hormones to do the same. Therefore, if you're considering menstrual management you need to understand how the hormones involved in the menstrual period work.

Five hormones play a role in regulating your menstrual period:

✳ *Gonadotropin-releasing hormone (GnRH).* GnRH is the "supervisor" hormone. It's in charge of all the other hormones involved with your period. GnRH is released from the brain, a little bit at a time, from an area called the hypothalamus. It controls the production and release of follicle-stimulating hormone (FSH) and luteinizing hormone (LH).

✳ *Follicle-stimulating hormone (FSH).* FSH is the supervisor's assistant. It is also released from the brain (from the area called the anterior pituitary). FSH regulates the production and action of two other hormones—estrogen and progesterone—and it is responsible for the production of a mature egg each month.

✳ *Luteinizing hormone (LH).* LH is another supervisor's assistant–type hormone released from the brain (from the anterior pituitary). It stimulates the production of estrogen, progesterone, and testosterone, and it is responsible for ovulation (the release of a mature egg from the ovary). Both FSH and LH influence the period—by controlling the release of estrogen and progesterone.

✳ *Estrogen.* Estrogen is one of the actual "worker hormones." It's secreted by the cells of the ovary (from the "granulosa" cells of the dominant follicle). Estrogen causes thickening of the lining of the uterus. It is also responsible for the development and maintenance of female secondary sexual characteristics (such as hair and fat distribution patterns and breast development).

✳ *Progesterone.* Progesterone is the other "worker hormone." It's secreted by the cells of the corpus luteum (what's left of the ovarian follicle after the egg is released). Progesterone maintains the lining of the uterus, before and after the fertilized egg implants. (Implantation is the burrowing of the fertilized egg into the lining of the uterus.) Progesterone also helps maintain female secondary sexual characteristics. Progesterone plays a key role in the menstrual period—its withdrawal initiates the period flow.

Once all the hormones begin to work together (feedback loops) everything begins to get a bit more complicated, especially when you consider that hormones don't just affect one another, they also act on many other body organs. For example, at the same time the estrogen acts on the ovary or the uterus, it also acts on bone, skin, the vagina, and the liver (estrogen-responsive tissues).

How does all this tie into menstrual management? When you use period control, the body hormone levels no longer fluctuate—they remain low and constant (they're said to be in a relative "steady" state). The levels of the synthetic hormones you're using are also fairly constant. How does all this affect you? Let's use estrogen as an example.

Rises and falls in hormone levels cause menstruation and prepare the body for pregnancy. If you're trying to become pregnant, you need these fluctuations. If you aren't trying to become pregnant, there's no biological reason for them. Actually, for many women, a steady level of hormone is actually beneficial. About 75–85 percent

---

✳ FAST FACT

Testosterone—yes, testosterone—is also produced by the ovaries, even though it is not directly involved in the menstrual cycle. In women, testosterone levels are much lower than in men. Although testosterone levels in women are difficult to measure accurately, the usual daily production rate in a woman is about 0.3 milligrams per day, while in a man it's 3.0 milligrams per day. In women, only about 2 percent of the total circulating testosterone is active; the rest is bound to a protein called

---

sex hormone–binding globulin (SHBG). Some hormonal birth control methods, like the Pill, increase SHBG, which means more testosterone will be bound and less free hormone will be available. By decreasing the amount of free testosterone, Pill use is able to help women with acne, excess hair growth (hirsutism), and polycystic ovarian syndrome (PCOS).

In men, testosterone determines a man's secondary sexual characteristics (larger muscle mass, deeper voice, hair distribution pattern) and its levels also have a direct influence on the man's sexual drive (libido)—a low testosterone level means a low sex drive.

This is not necessarily the case in women. For women, testosterone levels don't determine sex drive; factors such as current health, physical and social environment, cultural and educational background, past sexual experiences, relationships with partners, and estrogen levels play a role. There's no such thing as a set testosterone level above which women are "all set to go," nor is there a level below which women just can't get in the mood.

For example, a group of women whose sexual function was impaired (the women reported feeling less sexual excitement and also had lower testosterone levels) was given testosterone to raise its overall level. The increased hormone levels influenced the "mechanical" (physiological) aspects of sexual function (blood rushed to the vagina), but the women reported no change in their sexual excitement. In other studies, some women who use the Pill (and therefore have a decreased amount of free testosterone) reported increased sexual thoughts, whereas some women reported that they had reduced sexual thoughts while on the Pill. The shots (like Depo-Provera and Lunelle) rarely cause a loss of sexual desire, while women who use the implant method (like Norplant) were slightly more likely to experience mood disturbances.

The bottom line: if you experience a decreased sexual drive while using a hormonal method of birth control, first try to identify any other possible problems (like your general health, stress, your partner relationship). If you're sure it's none of those, changing your hormonal method of birth control (for example switching from the Pill to the skin patch) or stopping its use entirely might help.

of menstruating women experience some degree of premenstrual or menstrual problems, like painful periods, headaches, heavy bleeding, nausea, bloating, and breast tenderness. These problems are caused by changing hormone levels.

Women who use the Pill for birth control and who have a monthly fake period experience fewer period-related problems than do menstruating women, whose hormone levels vary throughout the month. One study found that 41 percent of women on the Pill reported that their menstrual-related problems improved, while 43 percent of women reported an overall quality-of-life improvement. However, this group is not entirely problem free. For one week each month, during the fake period, hormone levels still fluctuate. That's the week during which most of these women experience problems. Seventy-two percent of the women in the aforementioned study reported experiencing painful periods (dysmenorrhea), and 70 percent reported headaches.

For women practicing menstrual management, the severity of these problems is further decreased. Among them, they have typically only one week of hormonal fluctuation every six weeks to three months. In one study, 86 percent of women reported improvement in menstrual problems, and 94 percent reported overall quality-of-life improvement. Another study that compared problems like cramping, headaches, and bleeding in a birth control group and a menstrual management group found that the women in the menstrual management group had significantly fewer problems. Finally, in yet another study, 74 percent of women using menstrual management reported improvement both of original symptoms (painful periods, migraines, heavy bleeding) and in quality of life, as well as a high degree of satisfaction.

Bottom line: if you aren't trying to have a baby, the scientific consensus is that there is *"no apparent advantage provided by the wide fluctuation in the levels of estrogen that are characteristic of the [menstrual] ovarian cycle."* And the same is true when it comes to estrogen's far-reaching actions: keeping estrogen levels steady, as happens when you use birth or period control, doesn't have a negative impact on other body organs.

Your Monthly Cycle and Its Secrets

During the childbearing years, women have a menstrual period each month.

✳ DEFINITION

Theoretically, the "childbearing" years are considered to be ages 15 to 44. Of course, in reality it's possible to have a child at 14 or 48, but overall, most women have children when they're between 15 and 44 years old.

This means women spend over thirty-five years of their lives having over 450 periods. This makes the period a major part of your life. And yet, despite its prominent place, the menstrual period is only a small part of the monthly cycle. Why is this cycle important for you to understand?

* You'll have a better appreciation of how your body works.

* You'll understand how and why the menstrual period happens.

* You'll be able to make an informed decision about using period control.

* You can anticipate your fertile intervals.

Characteristics of the Monthly Cycle

Let's first look at some of the main characteristics of the monthly cycle.

The monthly cycles start with the first ovulation (the release of a matured egg from the ovary) and the first period (menarche) at puberty, at around 12 to 13 years old for girls who live in industrialized societies. They stop once a woman reaches menopause at around 51 years old. The menopausal woman stops ovulating and stops having a period.

The length of this "monthly" cycle varies from woman to woman and, sometimes, even for the same woman. Usually, during the first five to seven years after a teenager's first period, the cycles are more irregular and the interval between them is longer than for cycles later in life. Typically, they become increasingly shorter and more regular. When a woman enters her forties, the cycles begin to lengthen again.

So what's considered normal? An average cycle length is 28 days, but anything between about 24 to 35 days is normal and is fairly consistent from month to month in any given woman. The period flow lasts anywhere from 4 to 6 days, causes an average total blood loss of 25–60 milliliters, and can be light, moderate, or heavy. Flow longer than 7 days and blood loss of more than 80 milliliters are considered abnormal.

Although only 10–15 percent of cycles last exactly 28 days, by convention the 28-day cycle is considered the "ideal" cycle. (This doesn't mean that if your cycle isn't exactly 28 days you've fallen short of the ideal or that there's something wrong with you.) The number 28 is just an average—in this cycle, ovulation happens exactly at the halfway mark of the cycle, on Day 14. (In other words, it makes the math simple.)

✻ FAST FACT

A common reason for irregular cycles is anovulation—when ovulation doesn't occur, and no egg is released from the ovary. Anovulatory cycles are more common in women younger than 20 and older than 40. Anovulation may be an occasional occurrence—the result of high stress—or it can be caused by something severe like brain trauma.

Also, by convention, the first day of bleeding is considered Day 1 of the cycle, the period days are Day 1 through 5 (in an ideal cycle the period lasts for 5 days), and the cycle ends on Day 28. How does this translate into real life if your cycle isn't 28 days? Let's use an example to illustrate.

Let's say your period starts on the tenth of this month, your bleeding lasts for 3 days, and your cycle length is 30 days. This means that the day the bleeding starts, the tenth of the month, is Day 1 of your cycle. The period flow days are Day 1 through Day 3, or the tenth through the twelfth of the month, and your cycle ends on Day 30, or the ninth of next month. (The following day, the tenth of the month, will mark the beginning of the next cycle, with the bleeding starting again.) (See figure 3.)

April 2004						
Su	Mo	Tu	We	Th	Fr	Sa
				1	2	3
4	5	6	7	8	9	*10* ***Day 1***
11	*12*	13	14	15	16	17
18	19	20	21	22	23	24
25	26	27	28	29	30	

May 2004						
Su	Mo	Tu	We	Th	Fr	Sa
						1
2	3	4	5	6	7	8
9 ***Day 30***	10	11	12	13	14	15
16	17	18	19	20	21	22
23	24	25	26	27	28	29
30						

Figure 3 The days of the monthly cycle.

What Happens during the Monthly Cycle

During the monthly cycle, under the influence of hormones, the ovary and the uterus undergo a series of changes. The end result of these changes is a body that's ready for pregnancy. If there's no pregnancy, the monthly cycle starts all over again.

Of course, all the events in the monthly cycle are interrelated and happen along a continuum. But, for the sake of our discussion, we'll divide the monthly cycle into two simultaneous sets of events: an ovarian cycle, which produces and matures eggs and provides early pregnancy support; and a uterine cycle, which prepares the womb for a possible pregnancy every month.

THE OVARIAN CYCLE AND FERTILITY

The ovarian cycle takes place in the ovary; it accounts for egg production and early pregnancy support. This cycle is the fertility component of the monthly cycle. There are several benefits to understanding it:

* You can track the start and the duration of your period.

* You can calculate the most fertile time of your cycle (ovulation day).

Since this is a book about menstrual management you might wonder, why bother learning about the ovarian cycle? If you understand what happens during this cycle, you understand one key feature of period control: the ovaries determine fertility, not your period. In other words, the presence or absence of a period isn't the sign of fertility; the presence or absence of ovulation is. Just be-

---

✳ FAST FACT

In humans, the body prepares for an eventual pregnancy in the absence of an actual fertilized egg. In most other species, the fertilized egg has to be present first, and only then does the body prepare for a pregnancy.

---

cause a woman is menstruating, that doesn't mean she is fertile. Similarly, a woman who isn't menstruating may be fertile. (We'll discuss this in more detail in chapter 3.)

The ovarian cycle has five phases. By convention, the first phase of the cycle, the menstrual one, comes last in this list. For simplicity, we'll use a 28-day cycle as a model.

1. Follicular (early and advanced): Day 6 to Day 13
2. Ovulation: Day 14
3. Luteal (early and advanced): Day 15 to Day 25
4. Premenstrual: Day 26 to Day 28
5. Menstrual: Day 1 to Day 5

The first two phases are the "egg production" part of the ovarian cycle.

1. Follicular phase: egg maturation

A number of follicles containing eggs start developing and one dominant follicle matures.

There is increased estrogen, which reaches a maximum level just before ovulation. Progesterone levels are low, as are levels of FSH and LH.

> ✳ **FAST FACT**
> Actually, every month about twenty ovarian follicles start to mature, but usually only one follicle (the "dominant" follicle) fully matures and releases its egg; the other nineteen follicles degenerate.

2. Ovulation phase: egg release

One mature egg (ovum) is released from the dominant follicle. This is not a dainty process; it's more like a volcanic eruption—the egg bursts forth from the ovary. Then the egg enters the fallopian tube and travels through it until it reaches the uterus. Or, if fertilization occurs, the egg unites with the sperm usually in the outer third of the tube.

There is a big increase in LH (the "LH surge") about thirty-six hours before ovulation, an abrupt decline in estrogen, a steady progesterone increase, and a significant FSH surge (less prominent than the LH surge).

The next phase of the ovarian cycle is the "early pregnancy support" part of the cycle—the ovary gets ready, just in case a pregnancy occurs.

3. Luteal phase: pregnancy support

Once the egg has left the ovary, what's left of the ovarian follicle becomes the yellow body (corpus luteum). Its main function is to produce and release the hormone progesterone. Progesterone is essential for the development and support of an early pregnancy.

At this stage, there is a gradual rise in estrogen (maximal secretion rates). The progesterone secretion remains high until the end of this phase. There's an abrupt fall in FSH and low LH (reasonably constant until just prior to the next ovulation).

4. Premenstrual phase: getting ready for the next cycle

If there's no pregnancy, the yellow body (corpus luteum) triggers its own death, since it's no longer needed. At the same time, the ovary starts to prepare for the next monthly cycle, by starting to recruit new follicles.

> ✳ **FAST FACT**
>
> If a woman becomes pregnant, the corpus luteum produces progesterone until the sixth or seventh week of pregnancy, when the placenta (afterbirth) takes over progesterone production.

Estrogen and progesterone decline dramatically. There is a modest, but significant, increase in FSH secretion. The LH level is low.

5. Menstrual phase: the period

The yellow body (corpus luteum), which has lost all its nutrients, becomes the white body (corpus albicans). It shrivels up and is reabsorbed by the body. Recruitment of follicles for the next cycle continues. Estrogen and progesterone are low. FSH levels continue to decline, and LH levels remain low.

THE UTERINE CYCLE

The uterine cycle represents the changes that take place in the uterus, more specifically in the lining of the uterine cavity (the endometrium), during the monthly cycle. This cycle might be called the "ready and able in case a pregnancy happens" cycle.

Understanding this cycle will help you understand period control. In particular, you'll be able to recognize one key point: the period is all about the future, not the past. In other words, the period isn't so much a failure signal (your body has failed to become pregnant) as it is a readiness signal (your body is ready and able to support a pregnancy).

The uterine cycle can be divided into five phases (again we will use a 28-day cycle as a model):

1. Proliferative: Day 6 to 13
2. Ovulation: Day 14
3. Secretory: Day 15 to 25
4. Ischemic: Day 26 to 28
5. Menstrual: Day 1 to 5

How to Calculate Your Ovulation Day

It's a good idea to get into the habit of tracking your period data—the start of your period, its length, and the estimated start date of your next period. In addition to being able to predict your ovulation day (the time when you are most fertile), this will also help you if you plan to use menstrual management.

For example, let's say you have a big event scheduled in six months and you want to avoid having your period at that time. Since the best time to start using period control is about three months in advance of your planned event, knowing the anticipated date of your period will enable you to plan the start of your menstrual management regimen. (More on that in chapter 5.)

In a 28-day cycle, ovulation happens on Day 14. But if your cycle isn't twenty-eight days long, that doesn't mean much for you. Luckily, the day of ovulation is remarkably constant from woman to woman, and you can calculate your probable ovulation day based on the length of your monthly cycle. Think of the monthly cycle as being divided into two intervals: preovulatory (the interval from the end of your period to ovulation) and postovulatory (the interval from ovulation to the start of your next period).

THE MONTHLY CYCLE

Preovulatory (varying length)	Ovulation	Postovulatory (14 days)

↓

Period			Period

The length of the preovulatory interval varies widely, while the length of the postovulatory interval tends to be constant, at fourteen days, regardless of how many days your cycle lasts. In other words, there's no consistent relationship between the end of a menstrual period and the subsequent ovulation; the preovulatory interval may be four days, seven days, or nine days. However, the time between ovulation and the start of the next period tends to be constant. Fourteen days after you ovulate, you will get your period (unless, of course, you get pregnant).

So, to track your cycle, mark the day your period starts. This is Day 1 of your cycle. Then count the number of days until your next period starts. This is your cycle length. Do this for three cycles in a row. (The reason you need at least three months is because cycle length is not always the same each month. After three months you should be able to determine your average cycle length.) When your fourth period starts, count forward from Day 1 the number of days in your cycle length and mark that date. This is the anticipated start day of your next period. Then, from the anticipated start day, count backward fourteen days. This is your presumptive ovulation day (the day when you are most fertile).

For example, let's say your cycle lasts 23 days and your best friend's lasts 30 days. Both of you will likely ovulate 14 days before your next menstrual period starts. For you, this means ovulation day is Day 9 of your cycle (23 − 14 = 9). For your friend, ovulation happens on Day 16 of her cycle (30 − 14 = 16).

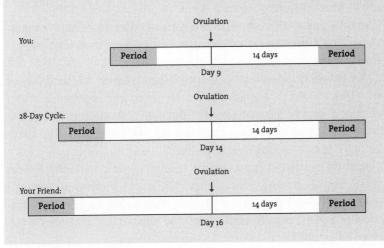

1. Proliferative phase: building up

The lining of the uterus (endometrium) starts to grow and there's a lot of activity in the tissue. The ovarian "granulosa" cells secrete increasing amounts of estrogen (in the form of estradiol), which stimulates the growth of the endometrium.

2. Ovulation phase: getting supplies

Drops (vacuoles) rich in nutrients (glycogen) start to form in the endometrium.

3. Secretory phase: fattening up

The uterine lining is completing its preparations for the possible implantation of a fertilized egg. The blood supply to the uterine lining becomes richer, the nutrient drops migrate toward the surface and release their content, and specialized changes in the uterine tissue (decidualization, described below) start.

At this point, the corpus luteum has begun to release progesterone. The combination of estrogen and progesterone causes *vascularization* (increased blood supply).

This is how decidualization works: When it comes to the ability of the uterus to accept a pregnancy, a fertilized egg, nutrients, and a rich blood supply are not enough. But don't blame the uterus; the "fault" rests mainly with the fertilized egg. This is because the fertilized egg has two unique characteristics.

First, the fertilized egg contains foreign genetic material. Sperm is made up of a man's genetic material, so it's viewed as "foreign tissue" by the woman's body. Because the fertilized egg is a combination of genetic material from both the woman and the man, it too is viewed as foreign tissue by the woman's body.

As long as the fertilized egg stays in its protective cocoon (zona pellucida) as it floats from the fallopian tube, where fertilization takes place, to the uterus, where implantation occurs, the "foreign tissue" issue isn't a problem. However, once the protective layer is removed and implantation starts, the egg's foreign tissue comes in direct contact with the woman's tissue. This poses a problem, because the woman's body has mechanisms in place to combat foreign tissue (as would occur in transplant rejection).

Second, the "technique" that a fertilized egg uses to burrow into the uterine wall is similar to the one cancer cells use to spread. To the body's defenses, it appears that the fertilized egg is aggressively invading the mother's uterine tissue. The woman's body is designed to stop this type of invasion.

In order for the uterus to accommodate a fertilized egg, the uterine tissue has to be able to receive the fertilized egg without rejecting it, and, once the egg has implanted, it must be able to limit its aggressive, tumorlike invasion. The way the uterus does that is: Close to the anticipated implantation time, the uterine tissue undergoes several highly specialized changes (decidualization)—cells build up a "wall" around themselves, and cells that regulate implantation are activated. Decidualization ensures that implantation goes off without a hitch.

4. Ischemic phase: slimming down

If a pregnancy doesn't happen, there is an abrupt decline in estrogen and progesterone levels. The drop in progesterone causes the top layer of the uterine lining to die. This, in turn, causes a tightening (vasoconstriction) of the uterine blood vessels, which leads to vessel destruction and bleeding into the tissue, and even more tissue death.

5. Menstrual phase: the period

The outer two-thirds of the uterine lining are shed. The period flow is made up of dead tissue, small pieces of endometrium, and blood. (Sometimes, you might see small blood clots in your menstrual flow. This is normal. If the clots become increasingly large, or there are a lot of them, consult your physician.) At the same time, rising

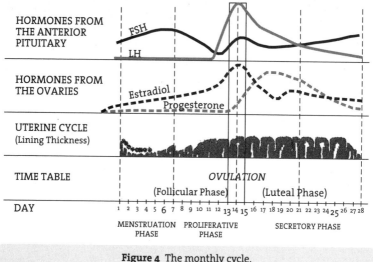

Figure 4 The monthly cycle.

estrogen levels cause the lining of the uterus (endometrium) to start to rebuild, in preparation for a new cycle.

WHY WE HAVE A MONTHLY CYCLE

In a nutshell, the reason we have a monthly cycle, and thus a period, is to prepare for a pregnancy. Unless you're planning a pregnancy, there's no known biological reason to have a monthly cycle. Of course, even if you don't want to become pregnant, you might wish to have one, but you don't need to. If having a period makes you feel feminine, beautiful, or sexy, then continuing to have a monthly period may be the right choice for you.

Throughout history, various theories have been presented to "explain" why we menstruate. Physicians in the third and fourth centuries B.C. believed that menstrual blood provided the raw material from which a baby was formed. Although we now know that theory isn't true, it managed to last for more than two thousand years!

By the early twentieth century, hormones and the heat cycle in animals were better understood. Scientists thought that menstrual

Hormones during the Monthly Cycle

FSH release is increased during the early follicular phase, and at ovulation there is a significant surge of FSH. During the luteal phase this level falls abruptly, and a small increase is noted during the premenstrual phase.

LH release is increased during the follicular phase, on about Day 9, which culminates with the highest levels ("LH surge") about thirty-six hours before ovulation. During the early luteal phase, the level gradually falls and remains low until just before the next cycle's ovulatory phase.

Estrogen levels are highest just before the preovulatory LH surge during the follicular phase. Immediately after or at ovulation there is an abrupt decrease in estrogen levels, then a gradual increase in the early luteal phase, with highest levels reached during the advanced luteal phase. Finally, during the premenstrual and menstrual phases estrogen levels decline significantly.

Progesterone levels are low during the follicular phase and start increasing steadily during ovulation. The levels remain high through the end of the luteal phase, decline rapidly during the premenstrual phase, and remain low during the menstrual phase.

bleeding was the same as the preovulatory bleeding of some animals. Today we know that this is also incorrect. The bleeding seen in animals (like dogs) isn't triggered by progesterone withdrawal and has a completely different trigger and mechanism (leakage of blood through intact vessels, called diapedesis)—it is not menstruation.

During the mid-1990s two important theories emerged. Beverly Strassman proposed that it was more efficient for the body to regularly shed the uterine lining than to keep it in a state of perpetual pregnancy readiness—the "energy conservation" theory.

Around the same time Colin Finn's theory explained the period as a necessary consequence of the unique evolutionary changes undergone by the fertilized egg (*trophoblast* invasion). Because the lining of the uterus has to commit itself to a "pregnancy" fate before a fertilized egg arrives, if there's no implantation, this specialized lining has to be shed to allow for the possibility of future pregnancies.

Finally in 1993, Margie Profet suggested that the period's function was to fight off the infections carried into a woman's uterus by the man's sperm. The press liked the "women vs. men" angle and popularized the theory. Some women found the idea intriguing and infused it with all sorts of social and cultural meanings. The widespread interpretation was that since menstrual bleeding is the uterus's way of fighting infection, stopping this bleeding artificially would be harmful to a woman's health.

Aside from the fact that neither the premise nor the interpretation of the actual facts used to support this theory are correct (we'll tackle this in chapter 3), the theory's predictions do not withstand scientific scrutiny. For example, we know that using the Pill, which artificially stops uterine bleeding, can actually protect the uterus from ascending infections (see page 45). So, if a woman heard about this theory, liked the way it sounded, and decided to base health decisions on its predictions, she might end up not taking the Pill and missing out on its health benefits. When it comes to period-related theories, always keep in mind that just because you like a theory, that doesn't make the theory good medical advice. For this reason, it's important when deciding whether menstrual management is right for you to first sift through the myths and facts about the period.

Chapter Two Bibliography

Cunningham GF, Gant NF, Leveno KJ, *et al*, eds. Internal generative organs. In: *Williams Obstetrics,* 21st ed. New York, NY: McGraw-Hill; 2001:39–40.

Ovarian Cysts

Teichmann AT, Brill K, Albring M, *et al.* The influence of the dose of ethinylestradiol in oral contraceptives on follicle growth. *Gynecol. Endocrinol.* 1995;9:299–305.

Brun JL, Le Touze O, Leng JJ. Medical and surgical treatment of functional ovarian cysts. *J Gynecol Obstet Biol Reprod (Paris)*. 2001 Nov; 30(Suppl) 1:S41–52.

Christensen JT, Boldsen JL, Westergaard JG. Functional ovarian cysts in premenopausal and gynecologically healthy women. *Contraception*. 2002 Sep;66(3): 153–7.

Lanes SF, Birmann B, Walker AM, *et al.* Oral contraceptive type and functional ovarian cysts. *Am. J. Obstet. Gynecol.* 1992;166:956–61.

Noncancerous Ovarian Tumors
Westhoff C, Britton JA, Gammon MD, *et al.* Oral contraceptive and benign ovarian tumors. *Am J Epidemiol.* 2000 Aug 1;152(3):242–6.

Polycystic Ovarian Syndrome (PCOS)
Guzick DS. Polycystic ovary syndrome. *Obstet Gynecol.* 2004 Jan;103(1): 181–93.

Cunningham GF, Gant NF, Leveno KJ, *et al*, eds. Internal generative organs. In: *Williams Obstetrics*, 21st ed. New York, NY: McGraw-Hill; 2001:51.

Johnson J, Canning J, Kaneko T, *et al.* Germline stem cells and follicular renewal in the postnatal mammalian ovary. *Nature.* 2004 Mar 11;428 (6979): 145–50.

Fibroids and Endometriosis
Child TJ, Tan SL. Endometriosis: aetiology, pathogenesis and treatment. *Drugs.* 2001;61(12): 1735–50.

Ling FW. Randomized controlled trial of depot leuprolide in patients with chronic pelvic pain and clinically suspected endometriosis. Pelvic Pain Study Group. *Obstet Gynecol.* 1999 Jan;93(1):51–8.

Sulak PJ. Should your patient be on extended-use OCs? *Contemp Ob Gyn.* 2003 Sep;48(9):35–46.

American College of Obstetrics and Gynecology. The use of hormonal contraception in women with coexisting medical conditions. *ACOG Practice Bulletin* No. 18. July 2000.

Speroff I, Glass RH, Kane G. Endometriosis. In: *Clinical Gynecologic Endocrinology and Infertility*, 6th ed. Baltimore, MD: Lippincot Williams & Williams; 1999:1063–4.

Testosterone

Vierhapper H, Nowotny P, Waldhäusl W. Determination of testosterone production rates in men and women using stable isotope/dilution and mass spectrometry. *J. Clin. Endocrinol. Metab.* 1997;82:1492–6.

Schreiner-Engel P, Schiavi RC, White D, *et al.* Low sexual desire in women: the role of reproductive hormones. *Horm Behav* 1989 Jun;23 (2):221–34.

van Santbrink EJ, Gianotten WL, Fauser BC. Androgens, well-being and libido in women. *Ned Tijdschr Geneeskd.* 2003 Sep 27;147(39): 1899–904.

Cutler WB, Garcia CR, Huggins GR, *et al.* Sexual behavior and steroid levels among gynecologically mature premenopausal women. *Fertil Steril.* 1986 Apr;45(4):496–502.

Apperloo MJ, Van Der Stege JG, Hoek A, *et al.* In the mood for sex: the value of androgens. *J Sex Marital Ther.* 2003 Mar–Apr;29(2):87–102; discussion 177–9.

Tutten A, Laan E, Panhuysen G, *et al.* Discrepancies between genital responses and subjective sexual function during testosterone substitution in women with hypothalamic amenorrhea. *Psychosom Med.* 1996 May–Jun;58(3):234–41.

Alexander GM, Sherwin BB, Bancroft J, *et al.* Testosterone and sexual behavior in oral contraceptive users and nonusers: a prospective study. *Horm Behav.* 1990 Sep;24(3):388–402.

Kaunitz AM, Wysocki SJ. Misperceptions about steroidal contraceptives and IUDs. In: *Dialogues in Contraception.* Winter 2002;7(7):3.

Bancroft J. Sexual effects of androgens in women: some theoretical considerations. *Fertil Steril.* 2002 Apr;77(Suppl 4):S55–9.

Bachmann G, Bancroft J, Braunstein G, *et al.* Female androgen insufficiency: the Princeton consensus statement on definition, classification, and assessment. *Fertil Steril.* 2002 Apr;77(4):660–5.

Feedback Loops

Sulak PJ. Creative use of oral contraceptives: perimenopause, menstrual disorders, premenstrual syndrome, and extended regimens. In: *Understanding Contraceptive Choices: The Patient's Perspective.* 2003 Nov:10–18.

Sulak PJ, Scow RD, Preece C, *et al*. Hormone withdrawal symptoms in oral contraceptive users. *Obstet Gynecol*. 2000;95:261–6.

Sulak PJ, Kuehl TJ, Ortiz M, *et al*. Acceptance of altering the standard 21-day/7-day oral contraceptive regimen to delay menses and reduce hormone withdrawal symptoms. *Am J Obstet Gynecol*. 2002;186(6): 1142–9.

Kwiecien M, Edelman A, Nichols MD, *et al*. Bleeding patterns and patient acceptability of standard or continuous dosing regimens of a low-dose oral contraceptive: a randomized trial. *Contraception*. 2003 Jan:67(1): 9–13.

Sulak PJ, Cressman BE, Waldrop E, *et al*. Extending the duration of active oral contraceptive pills to manage hormone withdrawal symptoms. *Obstet Gynecol*. 1997;89:179–183.

"... no apparent advantage ..."

Cunningham GF, Gant NF, Leveno KJ, *et al*, eds. Overview of human reproductive function. In: *Williams Obstetrics*. 21st ed. New York, NY: McGraw-Hill; 2001:18.

Your Monthly Cycle and Its Secrets

Oriel KA, Schrager S. Abnormal uterine bleeding. *Am Fam Physician*. Oct 1999;60(5):1371–81.

Cunningham GF, Gant NF, Leveno KJ, *et al*, eds. Clinical aspects of menstruation. In: *Williams Obstetrics*. 21st ed. New York, NY: McGraw-Hill; 2001:74–6.

Finn CA. Menstruation: a nonadaptive consequence of uterine evolution. *Q Rev Biol*. 1998 Jun;73(2):163–73.

Cunningham GF, Gant NF, Leveno KJ, *et al*, eds. Early human development. In: *Williams Obstetrics*. 21st ed. New York, NY: McGraw-Hill; 2001:89.

Cunningham GF, Gant NF, Leveno KJ, *et al*, eds. The Decidua. In: *Williams Obstetrics*. 21st ed. New York, NY: McGraw-Hill; 2001:78–82.

Cunningham GF, Gant NF, Leveno KJ, *et al*, eds. The endometrial cycle of ovulatory women. In: *Williams Obstetrics*. 21st ed. New York, NY: McGraw-Hill; 2001:71.

Strassmann B. The evolution of endometrial cycles and menstruation. *Quarterly Review of Biology*. 1996;71(2):181–220.

Finn CA. Why do women menstruate? Historical and evolutionary review. *Eur J Obs Gyn Rep Biol*. 1996;70:3–8.

Profet M. Menstruation as a defense against pathogens transported by sperm. *Quarterly Review of Biology*. 1993;68:335–81.

Hatcher RA, Trussell J, Stewart F, *et al. Contraceptive Technology* 17th ed. New York, NY: Ardent Media, Inc; 1998.

Panser LA, Phipps WR. Type of oral contraceptive in relation to acute initial episode of pelvic inflammatory disease. *Contraception*. 1991:43:91–9.

3

10 Myths about Monthlies
Common Misinformation about Your Period

* * *

For most of us, the first menstrual period marks the passage from girlhood to young adulthood. Long before we start having periods we hear all sorts of stories and bits of information—some more accurate than others—about this "welcome to womanhood." Ultimately, what the majority of women believe about the monthly period can be boiled down to three statements:

* Every month, year after year, from puberty until menopause, you'll have a menstrual period, with a few short interruptions for pregnancy and perhaps breastfeeding.

* Having a monthly period provides women with a wide range of health benefits.

* Since a monthly period can't hurt you, it's generally healthier to have a monthly period.

Well, guess what? Most of what you've been told about your menstrual period is wrong.

Before we look at what's fact and what's fiction, we need to clarify one point. How you feel about your period and what happens to your body during your period are two different things. For example, you may feel renewed and regenerated after having a period because you think your monthly period gives your body a rest. In reality, during your monthly period your body's activity is in full swing (more on this later). How you feel about your period is something unique to you and is always legitimate. Your explanation for this feeling, though, may not be.

It is important that you base your health decisions on accurate information. Unfortunately, getting accurate information isn't always easy. The amount of misinformation about the period and menstrual management is staggering. For example, even the FDA release on its approval of the first menstrual management pill, Seasonale, contained misinformation:

> *Under Seasonale's dosing regimen the number of expected* **menstrual periods** *that a woman usually experiences are reduced from once a month to about once every three months.* **As with the conventional 28-day regimen, women will have their period while taking the placebo tablets.** *[emphasis added]*

Women who use hormonal birth control, such as the Pill, don't have menstrual periods, they have fake periods (withdrawal bleeding). Technically, Seasonale doesn't reduce the number of menstrual periods—it changes the frequency of the fake period. (We'll discuss this fake period in detail in chapter 4.) So even this "official" information is misleading. It perpetuates the myth that the menstrual period and withdrawal bleeding are one and the same, and may lead women to believe that Seasonale reduces the number of periods and thus is less natural than traditional birth control. A woman who decides whether to use Seasonale because of this statement is making an important health and lifestyle decision based on inaccurate information.

This is just one myth among many. To deconstruct all the myths surrounding menstruation would require an entire book, so we'll touch only on the most common fallacies and misconceptions about the period and how they relate to menstrual management.

1. Having a monthly period is normal. *True, but . . .*

If you live in an industrialized society, and you're like most women, having a monthly period, for a lifetime total of about 450 periods, is normal. However, biologically speaking, it's unnatural.

Now, before I go any further, let me emphasize that "unnatural" does not mean bad or wrong. For example, it's unnatural for humans to fly because they don't have wings. Unassisted flight in humans is not the biological norm. However, not being able to fly isn't evil or an illness. The same applies to the menstrual period. Saying that a monthly menstrual period is not natural simply means a monthly period is not the biological norm.

> **✳ FAST FACT**
> Menstruation is very rare among animal species. Of the four thousand or so species of mammals, menstruation occurs only in the higher primates (humans and great apes), monkeys, elephant shrews, and two species of bats.

Determining the menstrual biological norm is not an easy task because in humans both nature and nurture play a role in a woman's menstrual frequency. So in order to get a clearer picture of the biological norm, we need to look at what happens in nature—a situation in which little, if any, nonbiological influences play a role, over many generations (tens of thousands of years.) To do this, we can look at animals like chimpanzees, our cave-dwelling human ancestors, and contemporary women who live in primitive societies away from the influences of the modern, industrialized world.

Because chimpanzees are one of the few species that menstruate, they can provide a good model for what constitutes normal menstruation uninfluenced by outside forces. Scientists have found that chimps living in the wild menstruate infrequently—every six years or so—because of repeated pregnancies and prolonged breast-feeding.

Scientists believe prehistoric women menstruated infrequently. Taking into account their life expectancy, the average number of children they had, nomadic patterns, and skeletal records, researchers have determined that our cave-dwelling ancestors had about fifty menstrual periods during their lifetime. This is not surprising, considering that most primitive women barely made it into their twenties.

But surely humans have evolved over thousands of years. Evolution alone must account for a change in frequency of menstruation, right? Not really. Until the last century or so (hardly a blink of an eye, in evolutionary time), women had only about 160 periods in their lifetime. Moreover, when scientists study contemporary women who live in societies far removed from the modern world, they don't observe a significant increase in the frequency of menstruation. Some of these societies include the !Kung, who are nomadic; the Dogon tribe of Mali, who don't use birth control; and the Hutterites of North America, a religious sect with 10.6 children per family. Overall, women in these societies experience their first period at around sixteen years of age, breastfeed their children for extended intervals (years), and have about 100 menstrual periods during their lifetime.

Compare this to the typical period pattern of modern women who live in an industrialized society and experience an average of 450 periods in their lifetime. Why are most women today menstruating more? Basically, changes in society have altered the frequency of menstruation. This is what I meant when I said that "nurture" also influences how often women menstruate.

Until recently women:

* *Had their first period in their late teens.* When people shifted from nomadic lifestyles to agricultural living, better nutrition and more food lowered the average age of the onset of menstruation to 12.5 years old (thus women menstruate for more total years).

* *Had a short life expectancy.* In ancient Rome the life expectancy was about 25 years. As recently as 1850, women lived for about 40 years. Compare this to 79.8 years, the average woman's life expectancy in the United States in 2001.

* *Lived in a society that depended on manual labor.* In order to ensure the survival of the species, early women had to have a lot of children because only a few survived. Today, due to a shift away from manual labor and toward better medicine, the replacement fertility rate (the rate needed to replace a population) is 2.1. Having fewer children means having more periods.

* *Had more children and breastfed almost continuously.* Women relied on breastfeeding to nourish their children, and they breastfed for much longer (years) and more often (forty-eight times per twelve hours). Today, lower infant mortality rates have decreased the number of pregnancies. Bottle-feeding is available as an alternative to breastfeeding, and even women who choose to breastfeed suckle the baby less frequently (about eight times in twenty-four hours). The less time a woman spends breastfeeding, the more menstrual periods she has.

* *Didn't have the ability to choose infertility.* Of course, the desire to prevent pregnancy has been around since the dawn of humanity—Egyptian women used crocodile-dung pessaries, and medieval ladies used diaphragm-like shields made of gold. The problem was that these methods were neither safe nor effective. However, with the invention of vulcanized rubber in 1839 and the subsequent development of reliable condoms, diaphragms, and cervical caps, as well as the revolutionary widespread use of the Pill after 1960, choosing temporary infertility became a viable option for women. Less time being pregnant means more time menstruating.

The bottom line: all of these societal factors influence modern women's biology and make it normal for women today to experience a monthly menstrual period, for a lifetime total of about 450 periods. Ironically, menstrual management allows modern women to return to a more natural state of prolonged menstrual suppression.

2. The monthly period reduces your risk of cancer. *False.*

Having a monthly period does not protect you from cancer. Actually, the opposite is true: women who use birth control and women who have lots of children—that is, women who have fewer periods—have greatly decreased risks of developing certain cancers.

UTERINE CANCER

Cancer of the uterus is the most common gynecological cancer. There were 38,300 uterine cancer cases and 6,600 deaths in 2000. For women who use the combination birth control pill, the risk of uterine cancer is reduced by 50 percent; women who use injectable birth control, like Depo-Provera, have as much as an 80 percent lower risk. (In fact, the shot is sometimes used as a treatment for metastatic uterine cancer—cancer that has spread beyond the uterus.) The cancer protection lasts for approximately fifteen to twenty years after you stop using the Pill. It's likely that all hormonal methods of birth control reduce uterine cancer risk to some degree; however, we have long-term studies only for the Pill and the shot, the two methods that have been around the longest.

Why the lower cancer risk? Most likely because the more menstrual cycles you have, the more times the uterine cells have to regenerate, and the more chances there are for abnormal or cancerous cells to form and go unnoticed in the uterine lining. Hormonal birth control and repeated pregnancy reduce the number of times the cells need to regenerate.

Although we'll discuss the relationship between each hormonal birth control method and cancer in later chapters, here's a quick summary for the other hormonal methods: Implants, such as Implanon, have no relationship to uterine cancer, while hormonal intrauterine devices (IUDs), such as Mirena, probably protect against it. No long-term information is available for the newer methods, like the skin patch and the vaginal ring.

OVARIAN CANCER

Ovarian cancer, which occurs in 1 out of 57 women, is the deadliest of all gynecological cancers and the fifth leading cause of cancer death in women in the United States. It is estimated that each year about 25,400 women in this country are diagnosed with ovarian cancer, and 14,300 die from it. Half of all women diagnosed with this disease die from it within five years, but early detection increases the odds of survival. For example, if the cancer is detected before it has spread beyond the ovary, more than 90 percent of women survive longer than five years. In contrast, if the detection happens once the cancer has advanced, only about 25 percent of women are alive at the five-year mark. Unfortunately, only about a quarter of cases are diagnosed early on.

> * **FAST FACT**
>
> Ovarian cancer is difficult to catch early because women usually don't have any symptoms. Even when symptoms are present, they're nonspecific—abdominal fullness. Adding to the difficulty is that there is no reliable test to screen for it.

The good news is that in women who use the combination pill, the risk of developing cancer of the ovary is reduced by 40–50 percent, and the protection lasts for thirty years after the last time the Pill is used. (Other hormonal methods, like the shot and implant, don't affect ovarian cancer risk, and information for the newer methods, like the skin patch and the vaginal ring, isn't yet available.) The most likely explanation of why this protective effect exists has to do with biological mistakes. During the monthly cycle, ovarian cells actively divide to repair and regenerate the ovarian follicles. Each time the cells divide, there is a possibility that an abnormality can occur and lead to cancer. The more periods you have, the more opportunities there are for mistakes to happen and to go undetected.

CERVICAL CANCER

In the United States, approximately 13,000 women develop cervical cancer and an estimated 4,100 women die from it each year. Cancer of the cervix is easily detectable—through a Pap smear, human papilloma virus (HPV) typing, and colposcopy. This cancer develops slowly and is relatively easy to treat. The survival rate for the preinvasive stage (carcinoma in situ) is greater than 95 percent, whereas for the invasive stage it's 70 percent for white women (56 percent for black women) at the five-year mark.

> ✳ **FAST FACT**
> Sexual behavior—early age at first intercourse and high number of sexual partners—is the major risk factor for developing cervical cancer. Minimizing this risk, together with consistently using a barrier method of birth control (which protects against STIs), makes sense.

For most women, neither using the Pill nor having a monthly period increases or reduces the risk of cervical cancer. However, HPV, the virus that causes genital warts, *is* a factor when it comes to cervical cancer. The majority of women who develop cervical cancer (94 percent of women with invasive cervical cancer, and 72 percent with carcinoma-in-situ [noninvasive cancer]) also test positive for HPV. In healthy women, there's no overall association between using the Pill and becoming HPV positive. In women infected with HPV, using the Pill for less than five years is not associated with an increased risk of cervical cancer; however, some studies suggest that, in women infected with HPV who had used the Pill for five to nine years, the risk of cervical cancer was increased. Additional research is under way and, although this is a small potential risk, you should be aware of it and discuss it with your physician.

BREAST CANCER

In the United States in 2001, approximately 192,200 cases of breast cancer were diagnosed, and an estimated 40,200 women died from the disease. Breast cancer is the second leading cause of cancer deaths (after lung cancer) in women. Most breast cancer cases (about 80 percent) occur in women over the age of 50.

Cases of breast cancer caused by genetic factors are due to gene mutations, like those on the BRCA-1 gene. A woman with a mutation on her BRCA-1 gene has an estimated 86 percent risk of developing breast cancer by the age of 70.

But some 95–98 percent of breast cancers are nongenetic, which puts all women at risk of developing it. The connection between breast cancer, menstruation, and the Pill has been studied and deliberated for years. Does the Pill increase your chances of developing breast cancer? Does menstruating protect you from it? We know that prolonged exposure to estrogen and/or progesterone can stimulate breast cancer cells to grow. (Not a good thing!) Both natural hormones (produced by the body during the monthly cycle) and man-made hormones (like the ones in hormonal birth control) have this effect on breast cancer cells. However, we also know that an increased number of monthly cycles increases your risk of breast cancer.

Studies have found that your risk is increased if you suffer from certain noncancerous breast diseases or if you menstruate frequently—for instance, your risk is increased if you give birth for the first time after age 30, have your first period at a very young age, or begin menopause late in life. It is believed that the increased number of menstrual cycles increases the breast cells' exposure to the estrogen made by the body. Because estrogen accelerates breast cell activity, there is a greater risk of random genetic errors that can lead to cancer.

So, how does the Pill fit into all of this? In 1996 the Collaborative Group on Hormonal Factors in Breast Cancer (CGHFBC) analyzed the data from 90 percent of the known studies about breast cancer and Pill use worldwide. The group's analysis found that there was a slightly increased relative risk of breast cancer diagnosis in current Pill users compared to never-users, but that the increased absolute risk due to Pill use is extremely small. For example, over one year, among 10,000 women aged 25 to 29 who use the

Pill, the number of breast cancer diagnoses would increase from 3.5 to 4.3. Actually, a comprehensive analysis of studies providing breast cancer risk estimates found that from age 35 to age 54, women who used the Pill had a slightly lower risk of breast cancer diagnosis when compared to nonusers. Current Pill users under the age of 35 have a slightly higher risk of being diagnosed with breast cancer. This higher rate of diagnosis could be due to these women going to the doctor to get birth control and thus being examined more often or it could be that the hormones in the Pill accelerate the growth of pre-existing cancers, thus allowing doctors to detect them at an earlier stage. In 1997 a very small genetic study (fourteen women), suggested that, for women with BRCA-1 or BRCA-2 gene mutations, Pill use might increase the risk of breast cancer. And a small historical cohort study in 2000 found that the old Pill brands (with a high estrogen dose) tripled the risk of breast cancer in women who had close relatives who had had the disease. However, the lower estrogen brands marketed after 1975 pose no excess risk. Finally, in 2002 a large U.S. population–based, case-controlled study called the Women's Contraceptive and Reproductive Experiences (CARE), which involved more than nine thousand women, found that for women aged 35 to 64 who use the Pill (both current and former users), there is no increased risk of breast cancer, even for Pill users with a family history of breast cancer.

The bottom line is that using the Pill has little or no effect on a woman's overall risk of breast cancer.

The progesterone-only shot, like Depo-Provera, doesn't increase risk the risk of breast cancer, and no relationship has been reported between implants, like Implanon, and breast cancer. The risk of the estrogen/progestin shot, like Lunelle, and that of the skin patch and vaginal ring aren't yet known.

COLORECTAL CANCER

In 2003 approximately 74,700 women were diagnosed with colorectal cancer in the United States. Although this type of cancer is the third most common cancer, both its incidence (the number of new cases that arise over a specific period of time) and its mortality rate are decreasing.

Having a monthly period has no effect on the risk of colorectal cancer. However, long-term use of the combination birth control pill may offer women protection against colorectal cancer. Results from the Nurses' Health Study, involving more than 1 million person-years (total number of study subjects and years studied) of follow-up, showed that among women who used the Pill for eight years or longer, the risk of developing colorectal cancer was 40 percent lower than the risk in women who never used the Pill.

✳ FAST FACT

Hormone replacement therapy (HRT) for postmenopausal women and Pill use in premenopausal women are very different. The findings of studies involving HRT apply only to women using HRT, not to women who use the Pill. If you're interested in HRT study findings, please visit www.tcoyp.com for information and resource listings.

---

3. Having a monthly period is good for your health and lowers your risk of heart attack. *False.*

Having a monthly period does not offer any special health advantages. In fact, for most women, outside of planning a pregnancy, there's no known medical benefit to having a monthly menstrual period. In healthy women, there are no conditions that are improved by losing blood on a regular basis. (Quite the contrary, cyclical blood loss can be detrimental.)

The only known instance in which people benefit from periodic blood loss is as a treatment for an inherited disease called hemochromatosis. Hemochromatosis results from excessive buildup of iron in various body organs. Too much iron can be toxic to our body. This condition is uncommon in women and occurs almost exclusively in people who have a genetic defect. Because we can absorb only about 10 percent of the iron we take in, unless you have this gene defect, you can't accumulate iron. Although both men and women can inherit the gene defect, men are five times more likely to develop the disease. Even in the small number of women with the gene defect, the chance of developing the disease is low because women tend to be chronically low on iron. If you have this genetic defect, you should use menstrual management with caution, if at all. Please talk to your doctor.

Having a monthly period doesn't reduce the risk of heart disease either. Heart disease is the number one killer of both women and men. More women die each year from heart disease than from the next seven leading causes of death combined. This very serious problem has numerous risk factors. Some you can't change:

* Age (the older you are, the higher the risk)

* Gender (men have a higher risk of heart attacks than do women in all age groups)

* Family history (you have a higher risk if a close blood relative already has heart disease)

* Race (black women have a higher risk of heart disease and stroke than do white women)

* Previous history of heart disease (if you've already had a heart attack or stroke, you're at a higher risk of having another one)

Others risk factors you can influence. These include: smoking, high blood cholesterol, high blood pressure, physical inactivity, excess weight, and high blood sugar (diabetes mellitus).

Overall, both menstruating women and postmenopausal women have a lower prevalence of heart disease, stroke, and heart attack risk than do men.

Interestingly, menstruating women have a lower risk of heart disease than postmenopausal women do. So how do we know that a monthly period doesn't protect against heart disease? Doctors have studied risk factors for healthy women who use hormonal birth control (menstrual suppression) and these women are not at an increased risk. They have also looked at the differences between menstruating and postmenopausal women to see if the lower risk in menstruating women could be related to menstruation.

Postmenopausal women tend to have higher body iron stores, less estrogen, and higher blood pressure than menstruating women. Studies have shown that higher iron levels aren't associated with an increased risk of heart attack. Recent trials have shown that increasing the levels of estrogen in postmenopausal women doesn't protect them from heart disease. Finally, higher blood pressure puts postmenopausal women at greater risk for heart disease. Having a monthly period doesn't affect blood pressure significantly—the hormonal fluctuations that take place during the monthly cycle are not associated with consistent changes in blood pressure or heart rate. So it is not menstruation that puts younger women at a lower risk for heart disease—it appears it's age and lower blood pressure.

4. Women need to have a monthly period to periodically clean out the uterus. *False.*

Having a monthly period doesn't flush out toxins. This myth originated around 400 B.C. Hippocrates, a famous ancient physician, and many of his peers believed that the body had "humors"—blood, bile, and lymph—and that an imbalance in any of them could cause disease. Thus, the cure for most disease was to flush these toxins out by bloodletting, vomiting, or purging. In fact, in A.D. 60, the first encyclopedia, *Natural History*, listed menstrual blood as a deadly poison.

Of course, today we have a much better understanding of how the body works, including the processes involved in toxin removal.

Normal waste is eliminated as urine and feces. The body fights toxins with antibodies in the blood and abscesses in tissues. The menstrual period doesn't rid the body of toxins—it simply expels bits of tissue from the uterus.

Moreover, the menstrual blood itself is not toxic—the lining of the uterus is sterile. Period blood is made up of cellular debris and liquefied clotted blood. There are no toxins in it. However, because blood is a good growth medium, if bacteria get into it they can grow and produce toxins. But this doesn't mean that menstrual blood itself is toxic.

As recently as 1993, Margie Profet, in the journal *Quarterly Review of Biology*, proposed a theory to explain why women have periods. In a nutshell, her theory says that the period's function is to protect a woman's uterus from men's bacteria-infested sperm. This idea is based on the observation that menstrual blood contains a lot of infection-fighting cells, like macrophages and other leukocytes. The theory proposes that the period solves the problem of the infected sperm by flooding the cavity of the uterus with these cells, which directly fight off the infection. In other words, this theory says that the menstrual period is a regular "disinfection" of the uterus.

Unfortunately, Profet misinterprets the presence of the infection-fighting cells in the period blood. The reason those cells are present in the uterine tissue and blood is because they play a crucial role in implantation (they're needed to limit the aggressive burrowing of the embryo into the uterus), as well as for the rebuilding phase of the endometrium, which starts during the menstrual period. Moreover, hormones, especially progesterone, not infection, are the trigger for these cells' action.

Furthermore, if this theory were valid, the following three statements (in italics), predicted by the theory, would be true.

There should be more infection (bacteria) in the uterus before the period than after. There's no evidence that there are more infectious agents in the uterus before the menstrual flow than immediately after it. In fact, a menstruating woman is more susceptible to various local infections than at any other time in her cycle. Moreover, menstrual blood is an excellent growth medium for bacteria.

Macrophages secrete a substance called vascular endothelial growth factor (VEGF), which helps new blood vessels to grow in the rebuilt uterine lining during menstruation. Leukocytes activate a group of enzymes called metalloproteinases (MMPs), which are needed for tissue remodeling; their activity is greatest during the first four days of the period.

The timing of menstruation should be related to the risk of infection from bacteria-laden sperm. Any bacteria-laden sperm entering the uterus soon after the period would have to wait for three weeks to be cleared away—plenty of time for an infection to develop. Also, pregnant and breastfeeding women, as well as postmenopausal women, wouldn't be able to fight the infection at all, because they don't menstruate.

The amount of menstrual bleeding should be greater in species with a promiscuous breeding system (frequent sex, multiple partners). Studies show that several nonpromiscuous primate species have copious menstrual bleeding.

The theory concludes with the suggestion that its hypothesis has medical implications, namely that *"artificially curtailing infection-induced uterine bleeding may be contraindicated."* In other words, stopping the period by artificial means (like when you use hormonal birth control) may promote uterine infection by undermining the body's natural infection-fighting mechanism.

As you can see, this theory has a lot of flaws, and the fact is, menstrual bleeding is not a disinfectant.

Another variation on this myth is the belief that a monthly period is always necessary in order to shed the lining of the uterus. Each month, under the influences of the fluctuating body hormone levels, the lining of the uterus thickens. The reason the lining thickens is to prepare for a possible pregnancy. If there is no reason for the body to prepare for pregnancy, the lining won't thicken. This is what happens when you use menstrual management. The lining remains thin. Because the lining of the uterus doesn't grow, there's no need to periodically shed it. Thus, the period becomes unnecessary during this time.

On a related note, there's no need to have a monthly period to relieve the "buildup" of natural body hormones because there's no such buildup. Throughout the monthly cycle the levels of hormones fluctuate. At the time of the period, there's no overall hormonal buildup; levels of most hormones are very low. The hormones in the Pill don't build up either. They are eliminated every twenty-four hours—that's why you have to take a pill every day, instead of once a week. (More on this in chapter 4.)

5. The monthly period allows the body to take a break from its normal activities. *False.*

Many women feel better both emotionally and intellectually during and after their periods. However, their bodies aren't at rest. In reality, the exact opposite is true. During the period, the body uses energy to narrow uterine blood vessels, shed the uterine lining, and repair and regenerate the lining. The uterus is not the only organ with a lot of activity during the period. In the ovary, new follicles with immature eggs are being recruited to start maturation.

The body is most at rest when both the ovarian and the uterine cycles remain in a low-functioning, steady state level—like when you use a hormonal method of birth control—and you don't have a menstrual period.

A lot of you have probably heard the common myth that it's a good idea to stop using hormonal methods of birth control, especially the Pill, after using them for a while, in order to give the body a break. Of course, this is not correct, and we'll discuss why in more detail in chapter 4.

6. The monthly period is a time of high sex drive. *False.*

In women, sexual drive is determined by many factors: past experiences, mood, hormone levels, and others. Studies looking at women's sex drive levels during the monthly cycle have not found that the menstrual period phase is an interval of increased sex drive. Of course, this doesn't mean that you might not feel the exact opposite. Every time you have a period, you may feel more in the mood, so to speak. A likely explanation for this is the placebo effect: most women think that it's not possible to get pregnant during their period so they're less inhibited and worried and more inclined to have sex, and this may be perceived as an "increased" sex drive.

> ✳ **FAST FACT**
> It is possible to become pregnant while having a period, although not very probable.

7. Having a monthly period "protects" you from becoming more like a man. *False.*

If you've been told ever since your first period that menstruating "makes you a woman," the thought of using menstrual management or hormonal birth control—having no monthly periods— might make you feel concerned. Relax. Biologically speaking, managing your period won't make you become more like a man.

A major difference between the sexes is their chromosomes. A chromosome is a unit of genetic material made up of *deoxyribonucleic acid* (DNA). Chromosomes define who we are as a species. Humans have forty-six chromosomes—twenty-two identical pairs, and a pair of "sex chromosomes": XX for women, XY for men. Having or not having a monthly period has no effect on your sex chromosomes. It doesn't change one of your Xs into a Y. Your female chromosomes are safe when it comes to menstrual management.

We can also differentiate between women and men based on the levels of "female" and "male" hormones—estrogen and testosterone. Both women and men produce estrogen and testosterone; however, reproductive-age women have more estrogen, while men have more testosterone. Both these hormones contribute to the development and maintenance of secondary sexual characteristics: muscle mass and fat deposit, hair distribution, breast development, etc. Using period control to skip the monthly period has no effect on the balance of these two hormones. In other words, when you use menstrual management your testosterone levels do not shoot up to equal a man's. (Actually, quite the opposite: the Pill tends to lower your testosterone level.) Nor does your estrogen level plummet. (On the contrary, instead of the periodic low levels women with monthly periods experience during the monthly cycle, women using menstrual management maintain a constant estrogen level.)

Another difference between women and men is reproductive organs. Women have ovaries, uteri, and vaginas. Men have testicles, prostates, and penises. Obviously, managing your period doesn't cause your uterus to vanish, nor do your ovaries or vagina mutate into new organs.

Similarly, if you use menstrual management, you don't become your grandmother. Women using hormonal birth control aren't menopausal. While it's true that women in neither group have a period, menopausal women stop menstruating because they have no more eggs and their ovaries stop working. Women using period management still have viable eggs and their ovaries still work perfectly fine; both the ovary and the eggs are simply on pause. Once you stop using menstrual management, your monthly cycles restart, as does your ability to conceive children. Also, pausing your monthly cycle, like when you use birth control or by having multiple pregnancies, doesn't hasten the onset of menopause.

8. Having a monthly period means that you will be able to have a baby.
False.

If you recall our discussion in chapter 2, the ovary and the egg determine fertility, while the uterus and the period determine pregnancy readiness. This might seem like a trivial difference, but it's not. If you menstruate but don't ovulate, you can't become pregnant. However, if you ovulate but don't menstruate, pregnancy is possible. This usually happens after a woman gives birth—the periods might take a while to return, but she could already be ovulating.

When you use a hormonal method of birth control, like the Pill, for either birth control or menstrual management, you're temporarily not fertile because you "pause" both ovulation and menstruation. (Since you're not interested in becoming pregnant at that particular time, you don't need to ovulate or menstruate.)

But what happens to your fertility once you stop using menstrual suppression?

For almost fifty years, women have used the Pill and scientists have studied what happens to fertility once women stop using it. This means we have nearly fifty years of information on how menstrual suppression affects fertility. In chapter 5 and 6 we'll go over the details of each hormonal birth control method and the time it takes for fertility to return. For now, suffice it to say that years of research show that using the Pill for menstrual suppression doesn't negatively affect your fertility once you stop using it. In other words, the Pill doesn't impair fertility. Actually, it appears quite the contrary is true. A study of more than eight thousand women found that women who had used the Pill had an increased ability to become pregnant (compared to nonusers). Moreover, the longer the women used the Pill, the better their chances of conceiving within the first six months after they stopped using it.

9. The monthly period acts as a vital sign. *False.*

If you have regular monthly periods and suddenly stop having a period or experience irregular cycles, this could be a sign that something is wrong. You could have a hormonal problem with either your brain or your thyroid gland, or have a nonhormonal problem with your uterus. Or it could mean there's nothing wrong with you—just a normal shift in your period pattern, or maybe you're pregnant. Having a period isn't even an absolute indicator of fertility. For example, women who don't ovulate (anovulatory women) have periods but can't become pregnant. Compare this to the pulse, a true vital sign. If you no longer have a pulse, your heart has stopped beating.

Bottom line: while the menstrual period (or rather lack of it) can sometimes indicate that something is wrong, it's too nonspecific to be a vital sign. The monthly period can serve as a general indicator of an underlying health problem. However, while there's nothing unhealthy about deliberately suppressing your period, as you do when you use birth control or period control, you should consider that whatever "health" signs you might have drawn from the monthly cycle are no longer present.

✳ FAST FACT

One poll found that more than two-thirds of the women surveyed did not rely on their period as a "health" sign.

---

10. Having a monthly period is generally healthier for you. *It depends.*
Just because having a monthly period doesn't give you any health benefits, that doesn't mean the period is unhealthy. On the other hand, for quite a number of women, limiting their number of periods is healthier.

There are two general groups of menstruating women: those who don't experience any period-related problems and/or who don't have any medical problems that can be made worse by the period; and those who suffer from period-related problems and/or whose health condition can be aggravated by the monthly period.

Obviously, for women in the first group the monthly period doesn't cause any health problems. However, even for this group, limiting the number of periods may be beneficial. That's because, even for these women, the risk of ovarian and uterine cancer decreases when they have fewer periods.

For the second group, the monthly period is associated with period problems, like cramps, breast pain and discomfort, bloating, nausea, acne, and premenstrual syndrome (PMS), as well as more major problems (anemia, migraine headaches, heavy and painful bleeding, seizures, and endometriosis).

✳ **FAST FACT**

In the United States, painful periods are the single largest cause of lost days at work and school for women under twenty-five years of age.

One of the more severe problems caused by menstrual bleeding is anemia. In the United States about 7.8 million teenage girls and women suffer from iron deficiency, of which 3.3 million have a more severe form called iron-deficiency anemia. The main cause of iron-deficiency anemia in premenopausal women is blood lost during menses. Unfortunately, because most women have learned to live with chronic anemia, it is often dismissed as a trivial problem. However, anemia can lead to long-term health problems and even death.

✳ **FAST FACT**

The World Health Organization considers iron deficiency the number one nutritional disorder in the world. It affects more than 30 percent of the world's population—that's over 2 billion people—particularly women of reproductive age and preschool children. This disorder has an important economic impact because it diminishes the capability of affected women to work, and it diminishes both growth and learning in children.

Bleeding disorders, although not as widespread, also pose a unique problem for women. For the women who suffer from them, the most common complaint is heavy and prolonged menstrual bleeding. Not surprisingly, the quality of life for these women is negatively affected by the monthly period. One survey found that 47 percent of these women felt less productive, and 38 percent reported that they had to reduce work and other activities while having their period. Sadly, many women are unaware that they have a bleeding disorder and are often misdiagnosed.

> **✳ FAST FACT**
> Von Willebrand's disease is thought to be the most common inherited bleeding disorder. It affects about 3 percent of the U.S. population and is due to a missing blood-clotting factor. Both men and women can have this disease, but women tend to be most frequently misdiagnosed. If you have von Willebrand's disease and would like more information, visit this site: http://www.tcoyp.com.

There's little doubt that women with iron-deficiency anemia or von Willebrand's disease benefit from having less frequent or no menstrual periods. Even if you don't have either of these conditions, period control may make sense for you. For many women, limiting the number of periods—by either having repeated pregnancies or using menstrual management—is a healthier choice. To make your decision you'll want to weigh both the risks and the benefits of each choice. This includes the side effects of the drugs used for menstrual management. In later chapters we'll look at the advantages and disadvantages of these drugs. Since in this chapter we looked at the real menstrual period, let's spend sometime discussing withdrawal bleeding—the "fake period"—next.

Chapter Three Bibliography

FDA Approves Seasonale Oral Contraceptive. FDA Talk Paper T03-65 September 5, 2003.

Finn CA. Why do women menstruate? Historical and evolutionary review. *Eur J Obs Gyn Rep Biol.* 1996;70:3–8.

Eaton SB, Pike MC, Short RV, *et al*. Women's reproductive cancers in evolutionary context. *Q Rev Biol*. 1994; 69:353–67.

Strassmann BI. Menstrual cycling and breast cancer: an evolutionary perspective. *J Women's Health*. 1999 Mar; 8(2):193–202.

Parkin TG. *Demography and Roman Society*. Ancient Society and History. Baltimore, MD: Johns Hopkins University Press; 1992.

Historical Statistics of the United States: Colonial Times to 1975. 1960. U.S. Department of Commerce. Washington D.C.

Arias E, Smith BL. Deaths: Preliminary Data for 2001. *National Vital Statistics Reports*. March 2003; 51(5):2. http://usgovinfo.about.com/gi/dynamic/offsite.htm?zi=1/XJ&sdn=usgovinfo&zu=http%3A%2F%2Fwww.cdc.gov%2Fnchs%2Fdata%2Fnvsr%2Fnvsr51%2Fnvsr51_05.pdf. Accessed May 14, 2004.

Fertility of American Women: June 2000. U.S. Department of Commerce, Economics and Statistics Administration, U.S. Census Bureau. http://www.census.gov/prod/2001pubs/p20-543rv.pdf. Accessed May 14, 2004.

Cunningham GF, Gant NF, Leveno KJ, *et al*, eds. Overview of human reproductive function. In: *Williams Obstetrics*. 21st ed. New York, NY: McGraw-Hill; 2001:16–18.

Connell EB. Contraception in the prepill era. *Contraception*. 1999 Jan; 59(1 Suppl):7S–10S.

UTERINE CANCER

World Health Organization. Endometrial cancer and combined oral contraceptives: the WHO collaborative study of neoplasia and steroid contraceptives. *Int J Epidemiol*. 1988;17:263–9.

The Cancer and Steroid Hormone Study of the Centers for Disease Control and the National Institute of Child Health and Human Development. Combination oral contraceptive use and the risk of endometrial cancer. *JAMA*. 1987;257:796–800.

Schlesselman JJ. Risk of endometrial cancer in relation to use of combined oral contraceptives: a practitioner's guide to meta-analysis. *Hum Reprod*. 1997;12:1851–63.

Voigt LF, Deng Q, Weiss NS. Recency, duration, and progestin content of oral contraceptives in relation to the incidence of endometrial cancer (Washington, USA). *Cancer Causes and Control.* 1994;5: 227–33.

Weiderpass E, Adami HO, Baron JA, *et al.* Use of oral contraceptives and endometrial cancer risk (Sweden). *Cancer Causes and Control.* 1999; 10: 277–84.

Levi F, La Vecchia C, Gulie C, *et al.* Oral contraceptives and the risk of endometrial cancer. *Cancer Causes and Control.* 1991;2:99–103.

World Health Organization Depotmedroxyprogesterone acetate (DMPA) and risk of endometrial cancer: the WHO Collaborative Study of Neoplasia and Steroid Contraceptives. *Int J Cancer.* 1991;49:186–90.

Kaunitz AM. Injectable contraception: new and existing options. *Obstet Gynecol Clin North Am.* 2000;27:741–80.

International Collaborative Post-Marketing Surveillance of Norplant. Postmarketing surveillance of Norplant contraceptive implants: II. Nonreproductive health. *Contraception.* 2001;63:187–209.

Hubacher D, Grimes DA. Noncontraceptive health benefits of intrauterine devices: a systematic review. *Obstet Gynecol Surv.* 2002;57:120–8.

OVARIAN CANCER

Ovarian Cancer: Reducing the Burden. 2003 Program Fact Sheet. Centers for Disease Control and Prevention. http://www.cdc.gov/cancer/ovarian/about.htm. Accessed May 14, 2004.

Ness RB, Grisso JA, Klapper J, *et al,* and the SHARE Study Group. Risk of ovarian cancer in relation to estrogen and progestin dose and use characteristics of oral contraceptives. *Am J Epidemiol.* 2000;152:233–41.

The Cancer and Steroid Hormone Study of the Centers for Disease Control and the National Institute of Child Health and Human Development. The reduction in risk of ovarian cancer associated with oral contraceptive use. *N Eng J Med.* 1987;316:650–5.

Rosenberg L, Palmer JR, Zauber AG, *et al.* A case-control study of oral contraceptive use and invasive epithelial ovarian cancer. *Am J Epidemiol.* 1994;139:654–61.

Narod SA, Risch H, Moslehi R, *et al.* Oral contraceptives and the risk of hereditary ovarian cancer. *N Engl J Med.* 1998;339:424–8.

Burkman RT. Oral contraceptives: current status. *Clin Obstet Gynecol.* 2001;44:62–72.

Pike MC, Spicer DV. Hormonal contraception and chemoprevention of female cancers. *Endocr Relat Cancer*. 2000;7:73–83.

Zieman M. Benefits beyond contraception. *Female Patient*. 2002 Dec; 27(Suppl):S12–S18.

CERVICAL CANCER

Bren L. Cervical cancer screening. *FDA Consumer Magazine*. Jan–Feb 2004. http://www.fda.gov/fdac/features/2004/104_cancer.html. Accessed May 14, 2004.

Moreno V, Bosch FX, Munoz N, *et al*. Effect of oral contraceptives on risk of cervical cancer in women with human papillomavirus infection: the IARC multicentric case-control study. *Lancet*. 2002;359: 1085–92.

Green J, Berrington de Gonzalez A, Smith JS, *et al*. Human papillomavirus infection and use of oral contraceptives. *Br J Cancer*. 2003 Jun 2; 88(11):1713–20.

BREAST CANCER

Breast cancer data. American Cancer Society. Cancer Facts & Figures: 2001:5.

The Contraception Report. *The Contraception Report*. 2000;11:2–16.

Burkman RT, Speroff L. Oral contraceptives and breast cancer. In: *Dialogues in Contraception*. Winter 2002;7(7):5–7.

Collins JA. Hormonal contraception and breast cancer: accounting for age at diagnosis. *J Soc Obstet Gynaecol Can*. 1995;17:33–42.

Ursin G, Henderson BE, Haile RW, *et al*. Does oral contraceptive use increase the risk of breast cancer in women with BRCA1/BRCA2 mutations more than in other women? *Cancer Res*. 1997;57:3678–81.

Grabrick DM, Hartmann LC, Cerhan JR, *et al*. Risk of breast cancer with oral contraceptive use in women with a family history of breast cancer. *JAMA*. 2000;284:1791–8.

Marchbanks PA, McDonald JA, Wilson HG, *et al*. Oral contraceptives and the risk of breast cancer. *N Engl J Med*. 2002;346:2025–32.

The WHO Collaborative Study of Neoplasia and Steroid Contraceptives. Breast cancer and depot-medroxyprogesterone acetate: a multinational study. *Lancet*. 1991;338:833–8.

COLORECTAL CANCER

American Cancer Society. Cancer Facts & Figures: 2003:4.

Mertinez ME, Grodstein F, Giovannucci E, *et al*. A prospective study of reproductive factors, oral contraceptive use, and risk of colorectal cancer. *Cancer Epidemiol Biomarkers Prev.* 1997;6:1–5.

Health and Risk of Heart Attack

Westhoff C, Kaunitz AM. An overview of menstruation. *Female Patient.* 2002 Apr;27(Suppl):S4.

Cunningham GF, Gant NF, Leveno KJ, *et al*, eds. Overview of human reproductive function. In: *Williams Obstetrics.* 21st ed. New York, NY: McGraw-Hill; 2001: 18.

Hemochromatosis. NIH Publication No. 02-4621. August 2002.

American Heart Association. *Heart Disease and Stroke Statistics—2004 Update.* Dallas, TX: American Heart Association; 2003.

Tomas Abadal L. Cardiovascular risk in menopause: myth, paradox or reality. The importance of clinical observations vs. statistical data interpretation. *Rev Esp Cardiol.* 1999 Jul;52(7):463–6.

Sidney S, Siscovick DS, Petitti DB, *et al*. Myocardial infarction and use of low-dose oral contraceptives: a pooled analysis of two US studies. *Circulation.* 1998;98:1058–63.

Rosenberg L, Palmer JR, Rao RS, *et al*. Low-dose oral contraceptive use and the risk of myocardial infarction. *Arch Inter Med.* 2001;161: 1065–1070.

Schwartz SM, Petitti DB, Siscovick DS, *et al*. Stroke and use of low-dose oral contraceptives in young women: a pooled analysis of two US studies. *Stroke.* 1998;29:2277–84.

Westhoff C. Depot medroxyprogesterone acetate contraception: metabolic parameters and mood changes. *J Reprod Med.* 1996;41:401–6.

Kaunitz AM. Injectable contraception: new and existing options. *Obstet Gynecol Clin North Am.* 2000;27:741–80.

Sempos CT, Looker AC, Gillum RF. Iron and heart disease: the epidemiologic data. *Nutr Rev.* 1996 Mar;54(3):73–84.

Sempos CT, Looker AC, Gillum RF, *et al*. Body iron stores and the risk of coronary heart disease. *N Engl J Med.* 1994 Apr 21;330(16):1119–24.

Fox CJ, Cullen DJ, Knuiman MW, *et al*. Effects of body iron stores and haemochromatosis genotypes on coronary heart disease outcomes in the Busselton health study. *J Cardiovasc Risk*. 2002 Oct;9(5):287–93.

Auer J, Rammer M, Berent R, *et al*. Body iron stores and coronary atherosclerosis assessed by coronary angiography. *Nutr Metab Cardiovasc Dis*. 2002 Oct;12(5):285–90.

Anderson GL, Limacher M, Assaf AR, *et al*. Effects of conjugated equine estrogen in postmenopausal women with hysterectomy: the Women's Health Initiative randomized controlled trial. *JAMA*. 2004 Apr 14;291 (14):1701–12.

Dubey RK, Oparil S, Imthurn B, Jackson EK. Sex hormones and hypertension. *Cardiovasc Res*. 2002 Feb 15;53(3):688–708.

Hirshoren N, Tzoran I, Makrienko I, *et al*. Menstrual cycle effects on the neurohumoral and autonomic nervous systems regulating cardiovascular system. *J Clin Endocrinol Metab*. 2002 Apr;87(4):1569–75.

Casiglia E, Ginocchio G, Tikhonoff V, *et al*. Blood pressure and metabolic profile after surgical menopause: comparison with fertile and naturally-menopausal women. *J Human Hypertension*. 2000;14:799–805.

Clean Out the Uterus and Take a Break

Coutinho EM, Segal SJ. *Is Menstruation Obsolete?* New York, NY: Oxford University Press; 1999:18, 24, 40–4.

Profet M. Menstruation as a defense against pathogens transported by sperm. *Q Rev Biol*. 1993 Sep;68(3):335–86.

Cunningham GF, Gant NF, Leveno KJ, *et al*, eds. Overview of human reproductive function. In: *Williams Obstetrics*. 21st ed. New York, NY: McGraw-Hill; 2001:72.

Salamonsen LA, Lathbury LJ. Endometrial leukocytes and menstruation. *Hum Reprod Update*. 2000;6(1):16–27.

King A. Uterine leukocytes and decidualization. *Hum Reprod Update*. 2000;6(1):28–36.

Critchley HO, Jones RL, Lea RG, *et al*. Role of inflammatory mediators in human endometrium during progesterone withdrawal and early pregnancy. *J Clin Endocrinol Metab*. 1999 Jan;84(1) 240:240–8.

Salamonsen LA, Kovacs GT, Findlay JK. Current concepts of the mechanisms of menstruation. *Baillieres Best Pract Res Clin Obstet Gynaecol*. 1999 Jun;13(2):161–79.

Strassmann B. The evolution of endometrial cycles and menstruation. *Quarterly Review of Biology*. 1996;71(2):181–220.

Finn CA. The adaptive significance of menstruation. The meaning of menstruation. *Hum Reprod*. 1994 Jul;9(7):1202–4.

Period is a Time of High Sex Drive

Dennerstein L, Gotts G, Brown JB, *et al*. The relationship between the menstrual cycle and female sexual interest in women with PMS complaints and volunteers. *Psychoneuroendocrinology*. 1994;19(3): 293–304.

Slob AK, Ernste M, van der Werfften Bosch JJ. Menstrual cycle phase and sexual arousability in women. *Arch Sex Behav*. 1991 Dec;20(6): 567–77.

Meuwissen I, Over R. Sexual arousal across phases of the human menstrual cycle. *Arch Sex Behav*. 1992 Apr;21(2):101–19.

Period "Protects" You from Becoming More Like a Man

University of Southern California. History of USC Reproductive Endocrinology and Infertility Program. http://www.usc.edu/schools/medicine/departments/obstetrics_gynecology/clinical/ivf/history.html. Accessed May 15, 2004.

Menstrual Suppression and Fertility

Cunningham GF, Gant NF, Leveno KJ, *et al*, eds. Overview of human reproductive function. In: *Williams Obstetrics*. 21st ed. New York, NY: McGraw-Hill; 2001:1529.

Farrow A, Hull MG, Northstone K, *et al*. Prolonged use of oral contraception before a planned pregnancy is associated with a decrease risk of delayed conception. *Hum Reprod*. 2002 Oct;17(10):2754–61.

Period as Vital Sign

Oriel KA, Schrager S. Abnormal uterine bleeding. *Am Fam Physician*. Oct 1999;60(5):1371–81.

Choosing When to Menstruate: The Role of Extended Contraception. Association of Reproductive Health Professionals Harris Poll. July–August 2002.

Kauntiz AM. Menstruation: choosing whether . . . and when. *Contraception*. 2000 Dec;62(6):277–84.

Ylikorkala O, Dawood MY. New concepts in dysmenorrhea. *Am J Obstet Gynecol*. 1978;130:833–47.

Centers for Disease Control. Recommendations to prevent and control iron deficiency in the United States. *Morbidity and Mortality Weekly Report*, April 03, 1998 / 47(RR-3);1–36.

World Health Organization. National strategies for overcoming micronutrient malnutrition. Document A 45/3, 1992.

World Health Organization. Battling iron deficiency anaemia. September 03, 2003. http://www.who.int/nut/ida.htm. Accessed May 14, 2004.

Kadir RA, Sabin CA, Pollard D, *et al*. Quality of life during menstruation in patients with inherited bleeding disorders. *Haemophilia* 1998; 4(6):836–41.

4

The Big Sting

The Difference between Real and Fake Periods

* * *

If I tell you that you don't have a menstrual period when you use the Pill, you might say to yourself, "But wait a minute; I've used birth control pills for years, and I still get a period every month!" True, you still bleed every month, but when you use a hormonal method of birth control, you stop having menstrual periods. They are completely gone and completely unnecessary. Surprised? Let's take this one step at a time.

There are over eighty methods of birth control, belonging to seven distinct groups:

* Hormonal
* Nonsteroidal pill
* Intrauterine devices (IUDs)
* Barrier and spermicide
* Natural family planning
* Sterilization
* Emergency contraception

Each group works differently and can come in a variety of forms. In the hormonal group, for example, there are six types of methods:

1. Birth control pill
2. Skin patch
3. Vaginal ring
4. Shots
5. Implants
6. Hormone-releasing intrauterine devices (IUDs)*

All forms of hormonal birth control have three things in common:

1. They contain synthetic (man-made) hormones.
2. They can be used to protect against a pregnancy or to manage your period.
3. When you use these methods, regardless of the reason—pregnancy protection or period control—you no longer have menstrual periods.

Only the methods in the hormonal group (including the hormone-releasing IUDs) can be used to manage your period. And since this book is about menstrual management, we'll focus exclusively on hormonal methods. So, any reference to birth control or birth control methods, unless otherwise specified, means hormonal methods only. (Although the hormone-releasing intrauterine devices are part of the IUD group, since, they use the same types of synthetic hormones as the other five methods of hormonal birth control, we will include them in the hormonal group.)

Where Have All the Periods Gone?
Why You Don't Have a Menstrual Period
When You Use Hormonal Birth Control

When you use a hormonal method of birth control you no longer have menstrual periods. Why? Well, the short answer is because you don't need to.

Recall that the period is only a small part of the menstrual cycle—the part of the monthly cycle that takes place inside the uterus. At the start of the cycle, the lining of the uterus is thin; then it builds up and becomes thick; and, finally, at the end of the cycle, most of it is shed in the form of the menstrual period.

All these changes in the lining of the uterus are caused by the rise and fall of your body's hormone levels. Both the hormones that act locally on the lining (estrogen and progesterone), and the ones that control the local hormones (follicle-stimulating hormone, FSH; and luteinizing hormone, LH) play a role.

Birth control, however, relies on synthetic hormones—man-made versions of the estrogen and progesterone your body makes. When you use synthetic hormones, your body happily "takes credit" for the birth control hormones and uses them as its own. Because your body no longer needs to make its own hormones, there are no more ups and downs in the hormone levels. All these changes last as long as you use birth control.

When the body's hormones no longer fluctuate, the lining of the uterus stays thin throughout the month, so there's no need to shed part of it regularly. No shedding means no menstrual period.

> ✳ **FAST FACT**
>
> If you're between 15 and 44 years old and you're sexually active, the most likely reason for a missed period is pregnancy. So, before you start worrying about this or that disease, make sure you're not pregnant. Take two home pregnancy tests, 24 to 48 hours apart, and consult with your doctor.

Doesn't the Lack of a Period Mean That Something Might Be Wrong?
Abnormal vs. Normal

If you're using hormonal birth control, not having a period is normal. Here's one way to think of the difference between no period and no period while you're using birth control:

When you go out in the sun, you get a tan. The UV rays activate the skin's cells to release a dark pigment called melanin. If you don't tan when you're exposed to the sun it may mean that you're as tanned as you are ever going to be. Or it could mean that there is a problem; your skin cells may not be working properly. However, you also will not tan if you use sunscreen, which blocks the UV rays and makes the release of melanin unnecessary. Not getting a tan when you use sunscreen is normal and expected.

Now let's look at menstruation. Getting your period is a normal result of your body preparing for pregnancy. If you don't get your period, it could mean that you are pregnant, or it could mean that something is wrong. You may have a hormonal imbalance caused by a problem with your pituitary or thyroid gland, or something in the uterus (e.g., fibrous bands called *synechiae*) may be blocking the flow of blood. If, however, you use hormonal birth control, not having a period is as normal as not getting a tan when you're wearing sunscreen. The hormones in the birth control pause your body's preparation for pregnancy, and therefore, having a period is not necessary.

So, if you're not using birth control and you stop having periods, there could be a problem; not having periods while you're using birth control is normal.

If It's Not a Period, Then What Is It?
What Happens inside Your Body When
You Use Hormonal Birth Control

If you've ever used birth control pills, or know someone who has, you may already know that every month you have a few days of bleeding, just like a menstrual period. The medical term for this bleeding is withdrawal bleeding, but we'll call it the fake period.

> ✳ **FAST FACT**
>
> Most of the time when you read about birth control or even when you talk to your doctor about it, you'll notice that there's no mention of "withdrawal bleeding." Rather, the term "period" is used instead. This is done mostly for convenience or to save time.

Why is it called withdrawal bleeding? When you use birth control pills, you stop taking the Pill or take a placebo (hormone-free) pill for one week each month. The fake period is caused by the drop in synthetic hormones. In essence, you've "withdrawn" the synthetic hormones from your body. Hence the medical term withdrawal bleeding.

The fake period is an artificial event that has nothing to do with your menstrual period. Instead, the dosage of birth control is manipulated to cause some shedding of the uterine lining.

To better understand the difference between the menstrual period and the fake period, we can use the suntan example again.

Think of the tan you get at the beach and the tan you get from a bottle of tanning lotion. The end result is similar: a nice overall tan. The same is true for the real menstrual period and the fake one: each month you bleed for a number of days. The difference is in the process.

For the real tan, you don't need to do anything—if you're outside in the sun, you get a tan. The same is true with your menstrual period—you don't need to do anything and you have a period.

In contrast, you only get a nice, overall artificial tan if you use the tanning lotion, and if you use a certain amount. You can't just use any old lotion, nor is it enough to put only a drop on your nose. The same applies to the fake period. The only reason you get it is because you use hormonal birth control and because you use a certain amount of it. If you change the dosage, you won't have a monthly fake period.

✳ FAST FACT

Because the fake period is an artificial event, it tends to be lighter, shorter, more regular, and less painful than the menstrual period.

Contrary to popular belief, the reduction in synthetic hormones that triggers the fake period doesn't give your body a "hormone-free" week or a "hormone break." As soon as the synthetic hormones from the Pill are unavailable to it, your body revs up its own local hormone production and the levels of the body's control hormones start to fluctuate. The end result: withdrawing the synthetic hormones causes disruption in the uterine lining that, in turn, causes it to bleed. This bleeding is the fake period.

At the end of the pill-free week, when you start taking the synthetic hormones again, your body stops producing its own hormones, constant levels of hormones are maintained, and the sequence starts all over again.

The Other Type of Fake Bleeding:
Breakthrough Bleeding (BTB)

Breakthrough bleeding (BTB) is the occasional, irregular bleeding or spotting some women experience while using hormonal birth control. It is most common when you first start using a method,

THE DIFFERENCE BETWEEN THE FAKE PERIOD
AND BREAKTHROUGH BLEEDING (BTB)

	Fake Period (Withdrawal Bleeding)	Breakthrough Bleeding (BTB)
Timing	Scheduled, intentional, usually monthly, regular	No fixed schedule, unintentional, anytime between two successive fake periods.
Character	Light bleeding	Spotting, light bleeding
Duration	Two to four days	Hours to a few days

and it usually stops after the first two to three months of use. However, this isn't always the case. Whether you experience BTB will depend on the brand, method, and your body. Moreover, BTB can occur whether you're using birth control to prevent a pregnancy or to manage your period.

Like the fake period, BTB has nothing to do with the menstrual period. BTB is an artificial event caused by the amount of hormones in birth control. Think of BTB as an "adjustment"—the bleeding occurs because the body is adjusting to the synthetic hormone dosages in the birth control method. We'll cover this in more detail when we discuss the individual birth control methods. For now, the important thing to remember is that the fake period and BTB are not one and the same. The table above outlines some of the differences.

Practically, there are two important things you should remember about BTB. First, BTB causes no ill health effects. Second, it isn't a sign that something's wrong; it's just a nuisance.

> ✳ **FAST FACT**
> Breakthrough bleeding is one of the main reasons women stop taking birth control pills. To lessen the effect of BTB, take the pill at the same time each day or try a different pill brand.

Do We Need to Bleed?
Is There a Need for a Monthly Fake Period?

Logically, you'd think that if scientific progress came up with the fake period (it didn't, but more on that later), there must be some health advantages. But that's just not the case. There's no medical need to have a monthly fake period. It doesn't offer you any health benefits, nor does the lack of a monthly fake period cause any health problems.

No Health Benefits

Having a monthly fake period does not offer you any health benefits. On the contrary, every time you have a fake period you are more likely to experience a host of health problems, like pelvic pain, headaches, nausea or vomiting, bloating or swelling, and breast tenderness. Why? Because all these problems tend to be caused, or worsened, by the fluctuations in hormone levels that cause the fake period. Let's use one of these problems, menstrual headaches, to illustrate the concept.

> ✳ **FAST FACT**
>
> Migraine headaches affect more than twice as many women as men. In 60–70 percent of women, the headaches are related to the menstrual cycle. Menstrual headaches that occur from three days before the start of your period to two days afterward are called true *menstrual migraines*. The ones that occur from one week to three days before the start of your period are called *premenstrual migraines*.

Menstrual headaches are a classic example of a problem thought to be caused by cyclic hormone changes. Scientists suspect falling and/or low estrogen levels trigger these headaches. Either the estrogen made by your body or the synthetic estrogen found in birth control can be the culprit.

During the menstrual cycle, both your body's local and control hormones go up and down. For example, at the end of the menstrual period, your estrogen levels start going up, hit a peak about midcycle, and then decline sharply right before the start of the next period. Similarly, if you're taking hormonal birth control, your fake period is triggered by withdrawing the synthetic hormones. In particular, the level of synthetic estrogen goes down suddenly, before your own body can rev up to produce enough to replace it. In either case, the result can be menstrual headaches. This dip in hormones, whether natural or synthetic, is also responsible for a wide range of other "menstrual" and "premenstrual" health complaints.

> ✳ **FAST FACT**
> Only the monophasic brands of combination birth control pills have the same amount of synthetic hormones in each pill. Other types of brands have varying amounts of hormones. We'll discuss the various pill brands in detail in chapter 5.

Fake Periods and Health Problems

Both natural hormones and synthetic hormones have the potential to cause various health problems. And, whether you're dealing with natural or synthetic hormones, the risk for these problems rises when you increase the amount of hormones and the exposure time to these hormones.

Women have been using hormonal birth control methods, like the Pill, for decades so we know the health risks associated with using synthetic hormones and having a monthly fake period. But what happens when you use menstrual management, and have a fake period less often, like every three months? The good news is that you won't be exposing your body to accumulating amounts of synthetic hormone because your body eliminates the synthetic hormones on a regular basis. For example, it takes your body about twenty-four hours to eliminate the hormones in one birth control pill. (This is why you have to take a pill every day.) So, it doesn't matter if you take the pill every day for three weeks in a row, or three months. Your body still takes only about twenty-four hours to eliminate the amount of hormones in one pill.

However, when you have a fake period less frequently than once a month, say every three months, your body is exposed to the synthetic hormones in birth control for 23 percent longer. For example, if you have a monthly fake period your body is exposed to the synthetic hormones for twenty-one days in a row, followed by seven days off, each month. In contrast, when you have a fake period every three months, your body is exposed to the hormones for eighty-four days, followed by seven days off.

The question is, does this increased exposure translate into increased health problems? Although there are no specific long-term studies, there are long-term data on the safety of using increased doses. This, together with additional recent evidence, indicates that the answer is no—not having a monthly fake period does not cause any health problem. Research in three health issues associated with hormonal birth control—the risk of developing a blood clot, the risk of cancer of the uterus, and the return to fertility—all supports this finding.

BLOOD CLOTS

Numerous studies have shown that when you use hormonal methods of birth control, the synthetic hormones—estrogen in particular—can increase the risk of blood clots and its associated complication (thromboembolisms).

So, what happens to your risk of developing a blood clot if you are exposed to synthetic hormones continuously and no longer have a monthly fake period? The answer, based on all the available evidence, is: nothing—the risk is no greater than if you take them for birth control purposes. And this answer holds true whether you're using birth control that contains only one hormone, progesterone, or a combination of estrogen and progesterone.

How do we know? Women have used methods like the birth control shot (e.g., Depo-Provera) and implants (e.g., Norplant) for decades. These methods, which contain only progesterone, eliminate the fake period for months to years at a time. Neither studies of these methods nor clinical evidence have shown an increase in the risk of developing a blood clot.

Similarly, studies of women using extended combination pill regimens showed that these pills do not increase your risk of developing a blood clot. Two studies in 2001 that looked at extending the use of the combination pill from twenty-one days to twenty-three days found no changes in the indicators that would signal an increased risk of forming a blood cloth. And in 2003, a large study of women who had a fake period only once every three months (they used Seasonale for one year) found no increase in nonmenstrual side effects compared to women who had a monthly fake period. Also, one of the combination pill brands already available for birth control, Mircette, has twenty-six days of hormone pills, and only two days without hormones each month.

UTERINE CANCER

Studies have shown that when you use combination birth control methods (which have both estrogen and progesterone) and you have a monthly fake period, the synthetic hormones significantly reduce your risk of developing uterine cancer (see chapter 3). But what happens to your uterine cancer risk if you no longer have a monthly fake period? After all, you're prolonging your body's exposure to hormones, in particular to estrogen. And we know that too much estrogen can cause uterine cancer. How does this extra exposure impact your risk of uterine cancer?

It is quite likely that the protective advantages of the synthetic hormones seen with the monthly fake-period regimen also apply to this prolonged exposure, but more studies are needed before this can be confirmed.

For now, let's look at the results of a few studies showing that eliminating the monthly fake period doesn't increase the risk of uterine cancer.

From UNICAMP University School of Medicine:
A 1999 study of women who had been using a combination monthly shot continuously, for a mean of two years, looked at the effects of the synthetic hormones on the lining of the uterus. Some of the women had a fake period every month, while others had no fake period for two years. The study found that the synthetic hormones had no negative effect on the lining of the uterus in either group of women.

From Eastern Virginia Medical School:
A study that looked at a combination pill brand (Mircette) where the pill-free week was reduced to only two days, for thirteen and fourteen months continuously, also found no effect of the extended continuous synthetic hormone exposure on the lining of the uterus.

In the Journal Contraception:
A study of women who used a combination pill (Seasonale) that caused a fake period only once every three months found that not

having a monthly fake period had no effect on the lining of the uterus.

RETURN TO FERTILITY

When you use any method of birth control you cannot become pregnant. Once you stop using the method, your ability to become pregnant (your fertility) returns. How long it takes for your fertility to return depends on which method you use. For example, once you stop using the Pill, your fertility usually returns within one month, whereas once you stop using the shot, it takes several months.

Eliminating the monthly fake period does not appear to increase the time it takes your fertility to return once you stop using that method. For example, when women use a monthly combination birth control shot, some have a monthly fake period, while about 15 percent stop having it for months to years in a row. However, the return to fertility for both groups typically takes two to three months after the last shot. Also, clinical evidence has shown that women who used the combination pill to eliminate the monthly fake period didn't have problems becoming pregnant once they stopped using the pill.

What Were They Thinking?
Who Invented the Fake Period and Why

History, not health, holds the answer to why we have a monthly fake period when we use birth control. It turns out that scientists built in a fake period to appease politicians and the Catholic Church, as well as to help the new method gain acceptance with women.

FOR ACCEPTANCE AMONG POLITICIANS

The introduction of the birth control pill has had an enormous impact on women's lives. On an individual level, women can plan when to have children or to decide not to have them altogether. As a result, they have been able to more easily pursue education and join the workforce. Between 1960 and 1999 the percentage of women who completed four or more years of college nearly quadrupled— from 5.8 percent to 23.1 percent. Also, between 1960 and 1999 the rate of married women who join the workforce almost doubled—from 31.9 percent to 61.2 percent.

The scientists who developed the birth control pill anticipated some of these revolutionary changes. At the same time they knew that these changes would likely trigger politicians' regulatory reflexes. So they thought that building a fake period into the birth control pill would make it seem more natural, which, in turn, could reduce backlash from politicians. While this may seem odd today, it had historic precedent.

Although women have used birth control for thousands of years—at the time of the Roman Empire, a plant called Sylphion was used to prevent pregnancies—it wasn't until the 1830s that birth control came into widespread use. The invention of vulcanized rubber in 1839 allowed mass production of condoms, diaphragms, and cervical caps.

Unfortunately, once birth control became more easily available, politicians stepped into the fray. In 1873 Congress passed the Comstock Laws, which prohibited sending birth control information and devices through the mail because they were "obscene, lewd, and lascivious."

Forty years later not much had changed. A three-year U.S. military sexually transmitted disease (STI) prevention effort, which included the distribution of chemical prophylactics for World War I soldiers to apply to their genitals after sex, was halted. The new Secretary of the Navy, Josephus Daniels, a Woodrow Wilson appointee, wrote: "It is wicked to encourage and approve placing in the hands of the men an appliance which will lead them to think that they may indulge in practices which are not sanctioned by moral, military, or civil law, with impunity, and the use of which would tend to subvert and destroy the very foundations of our moral and Christian beliefs and teachings in regard to these sexual matters."

The end result? Between 1917 and 1919, 380,000 soldiers (or 1 in 11) were diagnosed with an STI. The army estimates that by the end of the war it had spent $50 million on treatment. It wasn't until the 1940s that the military reversed its policy and made condoms available to troops.

This Big Brother trend continued. Birth control was actually legally forbidden in the United States for a long time. However, the tide began to turn in 1965 when the U.S. Supreme Court, in *Griswold v. Connecticut*, struck down state laws that had made the use of birth control by married couples illegal. In 1972, in *Eisenstadt v. Baird*, the court granted unmarried women access to birth control.

FOR ACCEPTANCE BY THE CATHOLIC CHURCH

Scientists also hoped that building a fake period into birth control would help birth control gain the approval of the Catholic Church by making the Pill appear more natural.

There were two main reasons why the scientists focused on the Catholic religion. First, by the time the Pill came around, most of the other major religions had already approved the use of birth control (in the context of marital sex, of course). Protestant leaders began easing religious restrictions on using birth control in the 1930s. Similarly, Reform and Conservative Judaism approved the liberal use of birth control in the early 1930s. Islam also allows the use of most methods of birth control.

The second reason was that around the time the Pill was developed, the church's leadership was reevaluating its relationship with its followers. In general terms, Pope John XXIII wanted the church to be less dogmatic and more all-embracing of the common person. So in 1962 he convened the Second Vatican Council, a gathering of religious leaders and experts, to examine a number of issues, including birth control. Scientists were hopeful that this new openness signaled that the church was ready to allow the use of the Pill. Unfortunately, Pope John XXIII died in 1963 before he finished his work.

His successor, Pope Paul VI, was afraid that approving birth control would undermine the church's authority. In short, he did not want to concede that the Protestants had made the right decision several decades earlier. Consequently, he overruled the majority recommendation to sanction the use of the Pill, made by the council he had appointed to research the issue, and he issued the Humanae Vitae ("Of Human Life"), in which he "categorically reaffirmed the prohibition of contraception."

Surprisingly, despite the church's rejection, within two years after the Humanae Vitae was issued, studies showed that as many Catholic women used the Pill as non-Catholics. By 1970, two-thirds of all Catholic women (and three-quarters of those under age 30) were using the Pill and other birth control methods banned by the church. More recent data shows that 96 percent of all Catholic women have used a modern birth control method. Church attendance frequency does not appear to make a difference: 73.5 percent of Catholic women who attend church once a week or more use birth control compared to 75 percent of Catholic women who attend less often (monthly).

FOR ACCEPTANCE AMONG WOMEN

Scientists knew that gaining acceptance for revolutionary ideas can be difficult. So to help the Pill gain popularity among women, they adjusted the dosage so that the fake period would mimic the natural period.

While you may think that the scientists were overly cautious or patronizing, don't be so quick to judge. A little more than 100 years ago, the concept of cleanliness to prevent infection was not widely accepted either.

Surgeons operated in their street clothes and didn't even wash their hands before surgery. As a result, many pregnant women died after delivery because of an infection known at that time as "childbed fever" (puerperal fever). Sadly, the infection was spread by the very physicians and nurses who delivered the babies. Here is a contemporary description of several 1821 deliveries:

"*Dr. Campbell, of Edinburgh, states that in October, 1821, he assisted at the post-mortem examination* [autopsy—ed.] *of a patient who died with puerperal fever. He carried the pelvic viscera* [internal organs—ed.] *in his pocket to the class-room. The same evening he attended a woman in labor without previously changing his clothes; this patient died. The next morning he delivered a woman with the forceps; she died also, and of many others who were seized with the disease within a few weeks, three shared the same fate in succession."*

The result was if you gave birth 100 years ago, you had a 1 in 200 chance of dying from a pregnancy-related problem. Today, your risk is closer to 1 in 10,000 if you live in a developed country. But those improvements didn't come easily or quickly.

One of the first essays on the connection between cleanliness and death from infections in postpartum women was published in the United States in 1843, by Dr. Oliver Wendell Holmes. He urged surgeons to wash their hands and change their clothes in between patients. Initially, this idea was considered unbelievable, even silly, by both the medical community and society.

Changing that perception took more than twenty years. Despite a succession of reports—including one by Dr. Ignaz Philipp Semmelweis that showed that women giving birth who were attended by doctors who performed autopsies were four to five times more likely to die—sterile practices didn't become widespread until well after 1865.

The inventors of the Pill learned from medical history. When they introduced birth control pill in the 1960s, they reasoned that women would feel more comfortable using the Pill if they still had a monthly bleeding episode, similar to their monthly menstrual periods.

However, another reason scientists created a monthly fake period was to reassure women that they were not pregnant. Today, a pregnancy test is often as easy as a trip to the neighborhood drugstore. In the early 1960s, however, if a woman thought she was pregnant she had to wait at least two months, then she had to visit her doctor, who would collect her urine and send it to the lab. The urine was injected into a female rabbit, which was killed and dissected. If the rabbit's ovaries were swollen, that meant that the woman was pregnant. The tests were time-consuming, complex, and not very accurate. At the time, they were also a pretty good reason for building in a fake period.

Of course, today birth control pills are no longer a novel concept. In fact, currently in the United States, birth control pills are the most commonly used reversible method of birth control, with over 10 million women using them.

Although times have changed because of birth control, the way many women use the Pill hasn't, even though many of the reasons for having a monthly fake period—political, religious, and personal reassurance—are now obsolete.

Since a monthly fake period doesn't offer any health benefits, the decision to have it really comes down to personal preference—for women whose life circumstances or health permit a choice. If you feel more comfortable pretending to have a monthly period because of cultural influences or personal philosophy, you don't need to change a thing.

However, if you decide you'd like to eliminate the fake period, or if your daily life, job, or health circumstances require it, this book helps arm you with the knowledge you need to consult with your physician to devise a plan that works for you.

So, What's the Real Deal about Fake Periods?
Myths vs. Reality

Saying that your health can benefit from the monthly fake period is like saying the world's current energy needs can be solved by using the matter/antimatter propulsion system of the *Enterprise*, the spaceship from *Star Trek*. The difference is that when it comes to *Star Trek*, fantastic speculation is fun and harmless. When it comes to making decisions about your health, it can be downright dangerous.

For example, in the United States about 10 percent of menstruating teenage girls and women suffer from iron deficiency. This corresponds to about 7.8 million women with low iron levels, of which 3.3 million have a more severe form called iron-deficiency anemia. If you have iron-deficiency anemia and use hormonal birth control, thinking that a monthly fake period is healthy and natural, you will experience a needless repeated loss of blood that can put your life at risk.

Although, for most women, menstrual management isn't a matter of life and death, it is essential that all women have the complete

---

✳ FAST FACT

Having the right iron levels is important because iron helps in the transport of oxygen, which is needed for cell survival. Meat, poultry, fish, seafood, and beans are good sources of iron. To lower your chance of iron deficiency and anemia, make sure you consume the recommended daily allowance (RDA) of iron. For teenagers, that's about 15 mg; for reproductive-age women it's 18 mg (27 mg for pregnant women); and for postmenopausal women it's 8 mg. For more information, please visit www.tcoyp.com.

and correct information about period control. So let's take a little time to debunk some of the most common myths about the fake period.

Myth #1: Even when you use birth control pills, you still have monthly menstrual periods.

Once you start using hormonal birth control, such as the Pill, you stop having menstrual cycles and, thus, menstrual periods. This is normal and it lasts the entire time you use these methods. The fact that you do have a fake period when you use hormonal birth control does not mean that you have a menstrual period. The two are not equivalent and are not interchangeable. Not knowing or understanding this basic concept gives rise to even more misinformation, which can be detrimental to your health.

Myth #2: The scientists who developed the Pill designed the monthly fake period because they knew that it's healthier to have a monthly menstrual period.

When using hormonal birth control, having a monthly bleeding episode is not natural and it doesn't offer you any health benefits. In fact, it isn't even really a period. The fake period is an artificial event. The reasons for the existence of the fake period are "designer" ones—cultural, social, religious—not medical. In fact, having a monthly fake period can be detrimental to your health. Every time you have a fake period you are more likely to experience a host of health problems.

Myth #3: You shouldn't use menstrual management because you need to have a monthly period while using hormonal methods of birth control.

This myth doesn't hold up on a number of fronts: First, the only reason you *need* to have a menstrual period each month is if you plan to become pregnant. Second, when you use hormonal birth control methods you stop having menstrual periods and you can't become pregnant for the entire time. You no longer have a menstrual cycle. What you do have when you use these methods is a monthly fake period. The only reason you have a fake period every month is because of the particular dosage of birth control that you're taking. When you use menstrual management, all you are doing is changing the frequency of the monthly fake period, not that of the menstrual period. (More on this in chapter 5.)

Myth #4: Because using menstrual management is a recent trend, we don't know if the regimens used for it are safe.

Menstrual management isn't a new concept. As a matter of fact, doctors have used period control to manage lifestyle issues and to treat a host of medical problems, such as heavy periods, hirsutism (excessive hair growth), endometriosis pain, and seizures, for decades.

In other words, not only have physicians been using menstrual management for years but, in many instances, menstrual management is considered the standard of care. This means physicians are professionally and ethically expected to use it.

As discussed in chapter 1, one reason you may not have heard much about menstrual management is that this was, until recently, an off-label use. Fortunately, this has now changed: in September 2003 the FDA gave its official seal of approval to the on-label use of one product for menstrual management, Seasonale. Hopefully, this will start easing the information embargo, and you'll have more opportunities to learn about menstrual management.

There's no shortage of data when it comes to safety either. The regimens used for menstrual management have been studied since the 1970s. Here are just some of the recent findings:

From Texas A & M University College of Medicine:
A 1997 study looked at using the Pill continuously for six to twelve weeks—meaning the women had a fake period only every six to

twelve weeks. The study concluded that this period control regimen is safe and works well. In 74 percent of users, period-related problems, like painful periods, heavy period bleeding, premenstrual syndrome (PMS), and menstrual migraines, improved.

From the University of Washington School of Medicine:
A 2001 two-year study compared a traditional 28-day cycle, which results in a monthly fake period, with a 49-day one, which results in having a fake period every seven weeks. This study found that having a fake period once every seven weeks is safe and results in fewer bleeding days and less breakthrough bleeding (BTB).

In the Journal Obstetrics and Gynecology:
A 2003 study that looked at using a very low-dose pill (20 micrograms of estrogen), continuously for one year, also found positive results. In particular, the study found that women using this regimen had significantly less bleeding than did women with monthly fake periods. (Spotting was greater during the first three months for the continuous regimen group, but by the end of the study there was no difference between the two groups.) Not only was the bleeding reduced, but there were also no adverse changes in the lining of the uterus.

For most birth control methods, there's considerable experience with the regimens used for menstrual management. When you use methods like the shot (Depo-Provera) or the implant (Norplant) for pregnancy protection, you stop having menstrual periods and fake ones for years. For these methods, the birth control and period control regimens are identical and the safety of the birth control regimens is well established. (See chapter 7 for a detailed discussion of these methods' safety profiles.) In any case, it's important to talk to your doctor about menstrual management. He or she can help determine the right method and dosage. Often this is relatively easy. However, for newer methods, like the patch and the vaginal ring, more long-term studies are needed to establish the optimal period control regimen.

Myth #5: Women want to bleed every month because of cultural or societal pressures.

Both older and more recent studies on this subject reveal that most women don't want to bleed every month. Moreover, most women favor control over how often they have a period.

A 1999 survey found that a majority of women (about 70 percent) would eliminate periods completely or at least reduce the bleeding frequency to less than once per month. Breaking down the numbers for one age group, the preferred frequency of bleeding was: every three months (38.3 percent), never (21.8 percent), every six months (7.8 percent), and once a year (4.0 percent). The percentage of women who liked having a monthly bleeding episode was 26.2 percent, and 1.9 percent were not inclined to use the Pill.

In 2002, the Association of Reproductive Health Professionals (ARHP) commissioned a Harris poll that found that of 491 women aged 18 to 49, overall, 44 percent of them would prefer to never have a period and 28 percent would prefer having a period every three months. Twenty-nine percent preferred to have a monthly period.

Finally, a survey of women in China, South Africa, Nigeria, and Scotland found that most women would opt to bleed only once every three months, or not at all. The exception: a majority of Nigerian women who'd prefer to bleed monthly. Interestingly, these Nigerian women were also the ones most likely to consider using a birth control method that completely stopped monthly bleeding.

From all these results, it appears that the main factor preventing women from using menstrual management is lack of information. While researching this book, I ran a quick, informal online poll at Global Health Options, a health site that focuses on information about birth control. While the findings aren't a statistically accurate depiction of the U.S. population, they do offer some interesting insights.

When asked if they knew how to use birth control to manage their menstrual period, 36.3 percent of the women said yes, 49.5 percent said no, and 14.3 percent were not sure.

Based on the type of site and the poll question, we can make a few educated assumptions about the 181 people who responded to the poll. Because Global Health Options is a health site, we can assume that the typical poll participant is more health-oriented (they specifically looked up birth control information) and more motivated (they took the time to answer the poll) than the average. So the poll results are more likely to reflect a more informed and motivated sample.

The results show that a majority of respondents (63.8 percent) either don't know or aren't sure how to use birth control to manage their period. In addition, the poll question is not very specific and there's no way to verify that the people who answered yes actually knew what menstrual management is. This makes it more likely that the "yes" result is artificially inflated.

So, even in a sample of well-informed and motivated people, the majority aren't familiar with menstrual management. This allows us to make an educated guess that probably most people have even less knowledge than our sample group of how to use hormonal birth control to manage the menstrual period.

Now that we've covered both the real as well as the fake period in some detail, in the next two chapters we will discuss the methods used for menstrual management. This comprehensive review will help you make informed decisions about menstrual management that most benefit your unique circumstances.

Chapter Four Bibliography

Abnormal vs. Normal

Laufer MR, Floor AE, Parsons KE, *et al*. Hormone testing in women with adult-onset amenorrhea. *Gynecol Obstet Invest*. 1995;40:200.

Loucks AB, Vaitukaitis J, Cameron JL, *et al*. The reproductive system and exercise in women. *Med Sci Sports Exerc*. 1992;24:S288.

Warren MP, Voussoughian F, Geer EB, *et al*. Functional hypothalamic amenorrhea: hypoleptinemia and disordered eating. *J Clin Endocrinol Metab*. 1999;84:873.

van Heusden AM, Fauser BC. Activity of the pituitary-ovarian axis in the pill-free interval during use of low-dose combined oral contraceptives. *Contraception*. 1999 Apr;59(4):237–43.

Breakthrough Bleeding (BTB)

Hatcher RA, Guillebaud J. The pill: combined oral contraceptives. In: Hatcher RA, Trussell J, Stewart F, *et al. Contraceptive Technology*, 17th ed. New York, Ardent Media; 1998:405–66.

Miller C, Murtagh J. Combined oral contraception. *Australian Family Physician*. 1992 Dec;21(12):1787–8.

No Health Benefits

Sulak PJ, Scow RD, Preece C, *et al.* Hormone withdrawal symptoms in oral contraceptive users. *Obstet Gynecol*. 2000 Feb;95(2):26–6

Silberstein SD. Menstrual migraine. *J Womens Health Gend Based Med*. 1999 Sep;8(7):919–31

Silberstein SD. Sex hormones and headache. *Rev Neurol* (Paris). 2000; 156(Suppl 4):S30–41.

MacGregor A. Migraine associated with menstruation. *Funct Neurol*. 2000;15(Suppl) 3:143–53.

Silberstein SD. Hormone-related headache. *Med Clin North Am*. 2001 Jul; 85(4):1017–35.

Fake Periods and Health Problems

Carr BR, Ory H. Estrogen and progestin components of oral contraceptives: relationship to vascular disease. *Contraception*. 1997;55:267–72.

World Health Organization Collaborative Study of Cardiovascular Disease and Steroid Hormone Contraception. Cardiovascular disease and use of oral and injectable progestogen-only contraceptives and combined injectable contraceptives: results of an international, multicenter, case-control study. *Contraception*. 1998;57:315–24.

Cachrimanidou AC, Hellberg D, Nilsson S, *et al.* Long-interval treatment regimen with a desogestrel-containing oral contraceptive. *Contraception*. 1993 Sep;48(3):205–16.

Endrikat J, Klipping C, Gerlinger C, *et al.* A double-blind comparative study of the effects of a 23-day oral contraceptive regimen with 20 microg ethinyl estradiol and 75 microg gestodene and a 21-day regimen with 30 microg ethinyl estradiol and 75 microg gestodene on hemostatic variables, lipids, and carbohydrate metabolism. *Contraception.* 2001 Oct;64(4):235–41.

Endrikat J, Cronin M, Gerlinger C, *et al.* Open, multicenter comparison of efficacy, cycle control, and tolerability of a 23-day oral contraceptive regimen with 20 microg ethinyl estradiol and 75 microg gestodene and a 21-day regimen with 20 microg ethinyl estradiol and 150 microg desogestrel. *Contraception.* 2001 Sep;64(3):201–7.

Anderson FD, Hait H. A multicenter, randomized study of an extended cycle oral contraceptive. *Contraception.* 2003;68(2):89–96.

(See also chapter 3.)

(See chapter 3, under uterine cancer.)

From UNICAMP University School of Medicine

Bahamondes L, Maradiegue E, Diaz J, *et al.* Endometrial histology in long-term users of the once-a-month injectable contraceptive Cyclofem. *Adv Contracept.* 1999;15(1):1–7.

From Eastern Virginia Medical School

Archer DF. Endometrial histology during use of a low-dose estrogen-desogestrel oral contraceptive with a reduced hormone-free interval. *Contraception.* 1999 Sep;60(3):151–4.

In the Journal Contraception

Anderson FD, Hait H. A multicenter, randomized study of an extended cycle oral contraceptive. *Contraception.* 2003;68(2):89–96

Miller L, Hughes JP. Continuous combination oral contraceptive pills to eliminate withdrawal bleeding: a randomized trail. *Obstet Gynecol.* 2003;101:653–661.

Lunelle manufacturer's product label. Pharmacia and Upjohn Company. Revised July 2001.

Bassol S, Garza-Flores J. Review of ovulation return upon discontinuation of once-a-month injectable contraceptives. *Contraception.* 1994 May; 49(5):441–53.

Bassol S, Hernandez C, Nava MP, *et al*. A comparative study on the return to ovulation following chronic use of once-a-month injectable contraceptives. *Contraception*. 1995 May;51(5):307–11.

World Health Organization. A multicentred Phase III comparative clinical trial of depot-medroxyprogesterone acetate given three-monthly at doses of 100mg or 150mg: 2. The comparison of bleeding patterns. *Contraception*. 1987 Jun;35(6):591–610.

The Faculty Speaks: Questions & Answers. *Female Patient*. 2003 Dec;28 (Suppl):S24.

Who Invented the Fake Period and Why?

U.S. Census Bureau, Statistical Abstract of the United States: 2000 Education, p 157.

U.S. Census Bureau, Statistical Abstract of the United States: 2000 Labor Force, Employment, and Earnings, p 408.

Riddle JM, *Contraception and Abortion from the Ancient World to the Renaissance*. Cambridge, MA: Harvard University Press; 1994.

Connell EB. Contraception in the prepill era. *Contraception*. 1999 Jan;59 (1 Suppl):S 7–10.

Forty-second Congress. Sess. III. CH. 258. Sec. 2 1873.

Tone A. *Devices and Desires: A History of Contraceptives in America*. New York, NY: Hill & Wang Pub; June 2001:91–115.

Griswold v. Connecticut, 381 U.S. 479 (1965)

Eisenstadt v. Baird, 405 U.S. 438 (1972)

Mastroianni L, Donaldson P, Kane T, eds. *Developing New Contraceptives: Obstacles and Opportunities*. Washington, DC: National Academy Press; 1990:43–5.

Boonstra H. *Islam, Women and Family Planning: A Primer*. The Guttmacher Report. Dec 2001;4(6).

Coffey K. It's time to end the hypocrisy on birth control. *U.S. Catholic*. June 1998:63(6):24–6.

McClory R. *Turning Point: The Inside Story of the Papal Birth Control Commission, and How Humanae Vitae Changed the Life of Patty Crowley and the Future of the Church*. New York, NY: Crossroad/ Herder & Herder; 1997.

Swomley J. The Pope and the Pill. The Catholic Church's teaching against contraceptive birth control has "laid a heavy burden on" innumerable people. *Christian Social Action*, February 1998;11(2):12.

Pope Paul VI. Humanae Vitae. *L'Osservatore Romano*. Vatican, 1968.

Catholics for Contraception. http://www.cath4choice.org/nobandwidth/English/contraception/catholics.htm. Accessed May 13, 2004.

U.S. Dept. of Health and Human Services, National Center for Health Statistics. Hyattsville, MD. National Survey of Family Growth, Cycle V, 1995.

National Center for Health Statistics. William Mosher, PhD, personal communication.

Holmes O. *The Contagiousness of Puerperal Fever*. Vol. XXXVIII, Part 5. The Harvard Classics. New York: P.F. Collier & Son, 1909–14; Bartleby.com, 2001. www.bartleby.com/38/5/. Accessed May 11, 2004.

Calvin S. *Ethical Challenges of Maternal-Fetal Medicine Practice in the United States*. International Forum on Medical Ethics, Tokyo, Japan. October 28, 2000.

Fenster J. *Mavericks, Miracles, and Medicine: The Pioneers Who Risked Their Lives to Bring Medicine into the Modern Age*. New York, NY: Carroll & Graf; 2003:76–90.

Early Years—Our History. Johnson & Johnson. http://www.jnj.com/our_company/history/history_section_1.htm;jsessionid=QQN31IW214TJ0CQPCCGSZOYKB2IIQNSC. Accessed May 11, 2004.

U.S. Food and Drug Administration. Guidance for Over-the-Counter (OTC) Human Chorionic Gonadotropin (hCG) 510(k)s. Document issued on: July 22, 2000.

Piccinino LJ, Mosher WD. Trends in contraceptive use in the United States: 1982–1995. *Fam Plann Perspect*. 1998;30:4–10, 46.

1999 Ortho Birth Control Study. Raritan, NJ: Ortho-McNeil Pharmaceutical, Inc.

Potts M. Birth control methods in the United States. *Fam Plann Perspect*. 1988;20:288.

Myths vs. Reality

Looker AC, Dallman PR, Carroll MD, *et al*. Prevalence of iron deficiency in the United States. *JAMA*. 1997;277:973–6.

(See chapter 3 also.)

National Academy of Sciences. *Dietary Reference Intakes for Vitamin A, Vitamin K, Arsenic, Boron, Chromium, Copper, Iodine, Iron, Manganese, Molybdenum, Nickel, Silicon, Vanadium, and Zinc.* Washington, D.C.: National Academies Press; 2000.

Myth #4:

FDA Approves Seasonale Oral Contraceptive. FDA Talk Paper T03-65 September 5, 2003.

From Texas A & M University College of Medicine

Sulak PJ, Cressman BE, Waldrop E, *et al.* Extending the duration of active oral contraceptive pills to manage hormone withdrawal symptoms. *Obstet Gynecol.* 1997 Feb;89(2):179–83.

From the University of Washington School of Medicine

Miller L, Notter KM. Menstrual reduction with extended use of combination oral contraceptive pills: randomized controlled trial. *Obstet Gynecol.* 2001 Nov;98(5 Pt 1):771–8.

In the Journal Obstetrics and Gynecology

Miller L, Hughes JP. Continuous combination oral contraceptive pills to eliminate withdrawal bleeding: a randomized trial. *Obstet Gynecol.* 2003;101:653–61.

Sulak PJ, Kuehl TJ, Ortiz M, Shull BL. Acceptance of altering the standard 21-day/7-day oral contraceptive regimen to delay menses and reduce hormone withdrawal symptoms. *Am J Obstet Gynecol.* 2002 Jun;186 (6):1142–9.

FOR SHOTS AND IMPLANTS

Kaunitz AM. Long-acting contraceptive options. *Int J Fertil Menopausal Stud.* 1996;41:69–76.

Akhter H, Dunson TR, Amatya RN, *et al.* A five-year clinical evaluation of NORPLANT contraceptive subdermal implants in Bangladeshi acceptors. *Contraception.* 1993;47:569–82.

Croxatto HB, Urbancsek J, Massai R, *et al.* A multicenter efficacy and safety of the single contraceptive implant Implanon. *Hum Reprod.* 1999;14:976–81.
(See chapters 3 and 6.)

Myth #5:

Kornaat H, Geerdink MH, Klitsie JW. The acceptance of a 7-week cycle with a modern low-dose oral contraceptive (Minulet). *Contraception.* 1992 Feb;45(2):119–27.

den Tonkelar I, Oddens BJ. Preferred frequency and characteristics of menstrual bleeding in relation to reproductive status, oral contraceptive use, and hormone replacement therapy use. *Contraception.* 1999;59: 357–62.

Association of Reproductive Health Professionals. Extended regimen oral contraceptives. Harris Poll. June 14–17, 2002.

Glasier AF, Smith KB, Vanderspuy ZM, *et al.* Amenorrhea associated with contraception—an international study on acceptability. *Contraception.* 2003 Jan;67(1):1–8.

Global Health Options, online poll. http://www.g-h-o.co.uk/index.htm. Accessed April 16, 2004.

5

Common Menstrual Management Tools

The Combination Birth Control Pill,
the Skin Patch, and the Vaginal Ring

* * *

Richard, a forty-five-year-old truck driver, has a headache. He takes aspirin, and it goes away. A week later, he has a doctor's appointment. The doctor tells Richard to start taking aspirin regularly to decrease his risk of a heart attack. Richard does so without giving it a second thought. He knows aspirin has many different uses.

Althea, a religious thirty-two-year-old, is recently widowed. Althea's problem is uterine fibroids (noncancerous growths inside the uterus) that cause her to have very heavy periods. The same doctor recommends Althea start using the birth control pill. Althea is furious, confused, and mortified. How can her doctor even suggest she is having sex outside of marriage? Althea, like many other women, doesn't know a little secret about the Pill: it has more than one use, too.

The Pill can do far more for you than just offer pregnancy protection. Here are the established, nonpregnancy-related health benefits of using the Pill:

* Period control and all its associated benefits

* Decreased incidence of cancer of the uterus and ovaries

* Decreased incidence of pelvic inflammatory disease (PID)

* Decreased incidence of ectopic pregnancy

* Decreased incidence of functional ovarian cysts

* Decreased incidence of benign breast diseases (fibroadenomas/fibrocystic breast disease)

Here are a few of the emerging health benefits of using the Pill:

* Treatment of dysfunctional uterine bleeding (DUB)

* Protection against colorectal cancer

* Attaining and maintaining optimal bone mass

* Protection against postmenopausal hip fracture

And here are some of the things women believe about using the Pill:

* About ninety percent don't know that the Pill protects against ovarian cancer and bone loss (osteoporosis).

* Thirty percent believe Pill use increases ovarian cancer and heart problems.

* Forty-one percent believe that Pill use is associated with substantial health risks.

* Fifty-two percent can't name any non-birth-control-related health benefits of the Pill.

This gap between reality—the proven health benefits of hormonal birth control—and women's perceptions of hormonal contraceptives is troubling. For example, in the United States alone, more than 10 million women already routinely take one of the drugs used for menstrual management, namely the birth control pill. Yet, most take the Pill for pregnancy protection, completely unaware of its full potential. This means millions of women already on the Pill suffer needlessly from ailments such as migraines or mood swings simply because they don't know how to take advantage of all the benefits offered by Pill use. Moreover, women who don't already use the Pill (some because they're not sexually active; some because they are using a nonhormonal method of birth control), and who think all the Pill is good for is pregnancy protection, are deprived of the option to use the Pill for all its health benefits.

So, the Pill and the other methods of hormonal birth control offer many other benefits besides pregnancy protection. One of these is menstrual management. But is this group of drugs the only method of period control? Of course not. Generally speaking, the period can be controlled by two means:

* Hormonal methods, including drugs and breastfeeding

* Surgical methods

Through most of this chapter and all of the following one, we will concentrate on the hormonal birth control methods that can be used for menstrual management, as well as on surgical options. But let's take a moment first to review some of the other types of drugs that can be used to manage periods.

Gonadotropin-Releasing Hormone (GnRH) Agonists

Gonadotropin-releasing hormone (GnRH) is a hormone, produced in the brain, whose main function is to regulate the sex hormones (the sex hormones are the ones involved in reproduction and period control). Think of GnRH as the CEO of sex hormones—it "makes sure" an egg is released from the ovary each month and that you have a menstrual period.

A GnRH agonist is a man-made hormone that mimics the natural hormone. However, rather than periodically releasing a dose of GnRH, which results in a period, synthetic GnRH is released continuously. Taking a steady amount of GnRH agonist has the exact opposite effect of taking the natural hormone—it suppresses the monthly menstrual period.

GnRH agonists can be taken in many forms—nasal spray, implant under the skin, or a shot—and, depending on the brand, they are taken daily to once every twelve weeks. The advantages of using this type of drug are:

* Good period control

* No daily dosage required (for some brands)

* Possible protection of the ovaries from the toxic effects of chemotherapy (more studies are needed to confirm this)

The disadvantages of using GnRH drugs depend on the duration of use. The longer you use them, the higher the risk of side effects. These include:

* Menopausal symptoms

* Decreased bone density (osteopenia)

* No pregnancy protection

* Cost (for some brands)

As a rule, think of GnRH agonists as the "big guns" of menstrual management, best reserved for women who need to stop having periods for medical reasons.

GnRH Antagonists

GnRH antagonists are drugs whose actions are exactly the opposite of GnRH. Since GnRH is responsible for a monthly period, using a GnRH antagonist for period control seems logical. Although there haven't been many studies on using this group of drugs for period control, the prospects are promising. Their main advantage over the GnRH agonists appears to be the fact that once you stop using them, their effects wash away faster.

Danazol

Another type of drug used for period control is danazol, a synthetic steroid that was one of the first drugs used for menstrual management. Danazol works by suppressing the sex hormones. It comes in the form of a pill that is taken daily, and the dosage is up to 800 milligrams per day. Danazol's advantage is good period control. It's usually used in women with endometriosis and heavy periods. Its disadvantages are:

* Masculinizing effects

* Menopausal symptoms

* No pregnancy protection

* Cost (expensive at $100 per month)

Because of its side effects and because it doesn't offer advantages over other drugs, danazol tends to be a second-tier drug, used when the other drugs don't work.

Now that we've reviewed some of the other drugs used for period control, we'll spend the rest of this chapter, as well as the next, discussing the bread and butter of menstrual management drugs: the hormonal birth control methods.

Hormonal Methods of Menstrual Management

Different hormones in specific amounts can suppress menstruation. This occurs naturally when you are pregnant (see chapter 1) and when you breastfeed. After giving birth, most women do not ovulate and do not have menstrual periods in the months immediately after delivery (usually for the first six months after delivery). This is a natural process called *lactational amenorrhea*—the hormonal processes involved in breast milk production (lactation) cause the absence of periods (amenorrhea).

Synthetic hormones are equally effective when it comes to controlling your period. Hormonal birth control and other drugs have been used for decades to limit or completely stop menstruation for lifestyle or health reasons.

There are six types of hormonal birth control:

1. Birth control pill—combination and progestin-only
2. Skin patch (Ortho Evra)
3. Vaginal ring (NuvaRing)

4. Shots—progestin-only (Depo-Provera, Noristerat) and combination (Lunelle)
5. Implants (Jadelle, Implanon)
6. Hormone-releasing intrauterine device (IUD) (Mirena)

To allow you to easily compare methods, we'll use a similar format for each section. First, there'll be an introduction to the method: what is it, who should and shouldn't use it, and what are its advantages and disadvantages. Second, we'll go over regimens used for both birth control and menstrual management. Knowing this information allows you to switch quickly and easily from use for birth control to menstrual management. In most cases the difference between the two uses is relatively minor.

Which method you use depends on what you want to achieve and on the degree of control you want to have. In the first chapter, we mentioned that when you use hormonal methods of birth control to manage your period, the degree of control you have varies. The best way to think about it is in terms of active versus passive management.

All hormonal birth control methods allow you to decide whether you have a menstrual period. That's because once you start using any of these methods, you no longer have a menstrual period for the entire time you use them. What you do have is a fake period, usually at a monthly interval. (There are exceptions to this rule; please consult with your doctor.) This is where the degree of control, active versus passive management, comes into play.

When you actively manage your period, you use a regimen that allows you to control whether you have a fake period, how often you have it, and, more or less, how long and how heavy it is. Three hormonal methods (the combination birth control pill, the skin patch, and the vaginal ring) can be used for active period control. Active management is best for women who want to manage their period for lifestyle reasons, as well as for women who suffer from period-related problems or whose health is made worse by having either a real or a fake monthly period.

When you use a passive menstrual management method you bleed less frequently and have shorter and lighter bleeding, or even no bleeding at all. The problem is that you can't control the outcome—it's impossible to predict beforehand what your bleeding pattern will be. Methods used for passive period control are the progestin-only birth control pill, the shots, implants, and the hormone-releasing intrauterine device (IUD). (Actually, there is some crossover—the progestin-only pill can also be used for active management. We'll discuss this in detail in chapter 6.) Passive period control is often well suited to women with period-related problems or whose health is made worse by having either a real or a fake monthly period, and for those who can't or don't want to use the active management methods.

You'll want to pick the method that's best suited to your particular needs. As your needs change, so may your optimal method. The more familiar you are with the available options, the better decisions you can make.

The Combination Birth Control Pill

Birth control pills are the second most common method of birth control used by American women. The birth control pill became available in 1957, and many brands are now available worldwide. In most countries, a doctor's prescription is required to buy them. Birth control pills are also called oral contraceptives, or oral contraceptive pills (OCPs).

There are two types of birth control pills:

* Combination pill (two hormones)

* Progestin-only pill (one hormone)

Since the combination pill is the one most commonly used for active menstrual management, we'll discuss it here; we'll look at the progestin-only pill in the next chapter.

The combination pill (the Pill) has two hormones: estrogen and progestin. These synthetic hormones are similar to the natural estrogen and progesterone produced by our bodies.

Most combination pill brands have the same type of estrogen, called ethinyl estradiol (EE). The amount of estrogen in each pill is very small—it's usually measured in micrograms (mcg). Different pill brands have different EE amounts—from a high of 50 mcg in the older brands (mostly manufactured and used before 1975), to a low of 15 mcg in newer ones. Brands with 35 mcg EE and less (low dose and very low dose) are most common today. The other estrogen used in combination pills is mestranol.

In contrast to estrogen, the progestins in combination pills are of many types. These progestins are sometimes referred to as first- and second-generation (the older ones) and third-generation (the newer ones). The amount of progestin in each pill is also very small, and it's usually measured in milligrams (mg).

TYPES OF PROGESTINS USED IN COMBINATION BIRTH CONTROL PILLS

FIRST- AND SECOND-GENERATION
PROGESTINS

- Norethindrone (norethisterone)
- Lynestrenol
- Ethynodiol diacetate
- Norgestrel
- Levonorgestrel

THIRD-GENERATION
PROGESTINS

- Desogestrel
- Gestodene
- Norgestimate
- Drospirenone (a newer type of progestin)

Because different pill brands have different types of progestins, you can't directly compare the strength of the brands. In other words, if two brands have the same dose but different progestin types, the potency can vary widely. For example, 0.5 mg of levonorgestrel is equivalent to 1 mg of norgestrel.

Who Can Use Combination Birth Control Pills?

Whether you're fifteen or forty-five you can use combination pills, provided that you don't have any risk factors. One common myth is that the Pill will stunt a teen's growth. This is false. Height is determined at a girl's first period. Once the first period (menarche) occurs, the body's estrogen stimulates a bone event (epiphyseal closure); it's this bone event that determines height. The Pill is also not unhealthy for teens. For some young girls, the Pill actually benefits their health because it helps manage common period-related problems (painful, irregular periods), improves acne, and provides effective birth control.

That said, some women should use combination pills only in very close consultation with their doctor and, even then, with a great deal of caution.

Be careful:

* If you are postpartum and gave birth at least twenty-one days ago and are not breastfeeding.

* If you are obese.

* If you have mild headaches or migraines without auras or visual disturbances.

* If you have diabetes without any blood vessel–related complications.

* If you have gallbladder disease, like gallstones, or take drugs that affect liver enzymes.

* **If you had breast cancer more than five years ago or have a family history of breast cancer.** (However, recent studies have shown that women with a family history of breast cancer who use the current low-dose pill brands don't have an increased risk of breast cancer.)

* **If you have a history of abnormal Pap smears.** An abnormal Pap smear could be due to uterine cancer, and women with this type of cancer shouldn't use the Pill. So it's best to first determine the reason for the abnormal Pap before using the Pill.

* **If you are a light smoker over the age of 35.** Light smoking means less than fifteen cigarettes per day. However, if you take combination pills you should strongly consider not smoking at all. Smoking increases your risk of serious heart and blood vessel diseases, whether or not you use birth control.

Who Cannot Use Combination Pills?

You should not use combination pills if you have any of the following conditions:

* **Known or suspected pregnancy.**

* **An allergy to any of the Pill's components.**

* **Blood clotting abnormalities.** Don't use combination pills if you have a history of blood clotting problems or any risk factors for them. Some of these factors are: blood clots in the legs (thrombophlebitis and DVT) or lungs (pulmonary embolism), and prolonged bed rest after surgery.

* **History of stroke or heart disease.** You shouldn't use combination pills if you have a history of stroke or heart disease, or any risk factors for them. Risk factors include migraines, or other headaches with auras or visual disturbances, and coronary artery disease. The coronary arteries are the blood vessels that supply the heart.

* **Diabetes (certain types only).** If you have a history of diabetes for more than twenty years or if you have diabetes with kidney, eye, or other complications related to blood vessel damage, you shouldn't use combination pills.

* **Known or suspected uterine cancer or any other estrogen-dependent cancer.** Estrogen-dependent cancer means any type of cancer that can be made worse by the presence of estrogen. In general, cancers of the genital organs, like uterine cancer, are estrogen-dependent.

* **Abnormal genital bleeding (e.g., from the uterus or vagina).** Don't start using the Pill until the cause of the abnormal bleeding has been diagnosed and treated.

* **Known or suspected liver cancer or other liver diseases.** If you had jaundice during pregnancy or jaundice with prior combination pill use, you should not use combination pills.

* **If you are a heavy smoker over the age of 35.** Heavy smokers smoke fifteen or more cigarettes per day. Because smoking increases the risk of serious heart and blood vessel disease for everyone, you should strongly consider not smoking at all.

Advantages of Using the Combination Birth Control Pill

You can use the Pill to manage your menstrual period. Lifestyle advantages can include convenience and increased productivity, while health-care reasons deal with improving a period problem or treating a medical condition. In addition to lowering the number of yearly periods and reducing the frequency of common period-related problems like cramping, managing the period offers women a way to lessen or even treat a number of medical conditions related to periods. Here are some examples:

* *Period disorders.* Women who suffer from either real or fake period–related problems can benefit from using the Pill and menstrual management. For example, if you have irregular menstrual

cycles, or heavy or painful periods, you can use this method to regulate the cycles and decrease the amount of bleeding. You can also greatly reduce the premenstrual syndrome (PMS) associated with the hormone-free or placebo week.

✳ FAST FACT

PMS includes both physical and behavioral problems like bloating, breast tenderness, swelling of hands and feet, headache, depressed mood, anxiety or tension, angry outbursts, irritability, decreased interest in usual activities, and poor concentration. These symptoms are severe enough to interfere with normal, day-to-day activities, tend to start during the last one or two weeks of the menstrual cycle, and disappear by the end of the period. Additionally, about 1–8 percent of reproductive-age women suffer from a more severe period-related problem called premenstrual dysphoric disorder (PMDD). For more information about PMDD, please visit www.tcoyp.com.

✳ *Anemia.* Iron-deficiency anemia is a serious, worldwide health problem, and women bear the brunt of it. If your period flow lasts five days or longer, is heavy, or you pass a large number of clots, it's likely you're anemic. Reducing or stopping the period blood loss replenishes the body's iron stores and improves the anemia.

✳ *Bleeding disorders.* Women who suffer from von Willebrand's disease or factor XI deficiency, or who are hemophilia carriers can benefit from the reduction in menstrual bleeding.

✳ *Endometriosis.* Having monthly periods, real or fake, tends to aggravate this health problem. Using menstrual management is helpful in treating endometriosis. (For more on endometriosis, see chapter 2.)

✳ *Uterine fibroids.* Uterine fibroids are associated with heavy bleeding, painful periods, and bowel and bladder problems (urinary frequency, constipation). Period control can decrease the amount of blood loss, so it's a good first-line management option. (For more on fibroids, see chapter 2.)

* *Functional ovarian cysts (noncancerous cysts).* Because the body's natural hormonal level fluctuations can cause functional ovarian cysts to form, using combination pills decreases the likelihood of these cysts forming.

* *Benign breast diseases.* Using the Pill can reduce the incidence of various noncancerous (benign) breast conditions.

* *Menstrual migraines.* Using menstrual management helps women who suffer from migraine headaches associated with the period.

* *Epilepsy/seizures.* In addition to having fewer period-related seizures, these women can benefit from using the Pill for menstrual management because of the increased pregnancy protection. (Antiseizure medications tend to reduce the Pill's birth control effectiveness.)

* *Asthma.*

The Pill has many other health benefits unrelated to its ability to prevent a pregnancy. Some of these benefits are:

* *Reduced risk of ovarian and uterine cancers.* If you use the Pill short-term (less than ten years) you reduce your risk of ovarian cancer by 40 percent. If you use it long-term (ten or more years) your risk is reduced by as much as 80 percent. In addition, this protection persists for at least nineteen years after you stop taking the pills. Using the Pill for five years halves your risk of uterine cancer. After twelve years of use, your risk reduction goes up to 72 percent. This protection persists for at least twenty years after you stop taking the Pill. (See chapter 3.)

* *Reduced acne.* Acne affects more than a quarter of women aged 15 to 44. Studies show that using the Pill significantly reduces both the total number of acne lesions as well as the num-

ber of inflammatory ones. In the United States only certain brands (*Ortho Tri-Cyclen*) are FDA-approved to be labeled for treating acne. Of course, other brands can help reduce acne, and labels on brands outside the United States reflect that.

* *Limited protection against pelvic inflammatory disease (PID).* Using the Pill has been associated with a reduction as great as 60 percent in a woman's risk of hospitalization for PID. (For more on PID, see chapter 2.)

* *Lowered risk of ectopic pregnancy.*

* *A positive effect on bone density.* The Pill has an overall positive effect on maintaining bone density. Not only does it not cause bone loss, but it also appears to actively prevent it. For example, studies in perimenopausal women have shown that using the Pill actually prevents bone degeneration. The Pill can also help teenagers whose estrogen levels are very low, due to excessive exercise or eating disorders, and young women in general to attain maximum bone density.

* *Improved hirsutism.* In a woman, hirsutism means excessive hair growth in a male pattern—on the chin, face, or chest. Combination pills can lessen the hormonal imbalance that causes this condition.

* *Improved rheumatoid arthritis.* So far, studies have found that using the Pill reduces a woman's risk of developing rheumatoid arthritis (RA) by 43 percent. This protection is more pronounced for RF-positive than for RF-negative RA. (More studies are needed to confirm this.)

* *Improved cholesterol and other lipid levels.*

Note: The skin patch (Ortho Evra) and the vaginal ring (Nuva-Ring) are much newer than the Pill. This means there are fewer studies and less clinical experience proving the general health benefits mentioned above. However, because the skin patch and the vaginal ring work on the same principle as the Pill, it's expected that using them will offer the same benefits. (Studies using the patch and the ring are under way to confirm this.)

Disadvantages of Using the Combination Birth Control Pill

Estrogen and progestin have a number of side effects. Below are the typical side effects you'd experience if you use the Pill for birth control.

Estrogen
* Nausea and vomiting (although the most common side effect, you can often control it by taking the Pill at bedtime or with a meal)

* Headaches and dizziness

* Depression (older brands containing 50 micrograms of estrogen)

* Breast tenderness and enlargement

* Increased cervical secretions

* Increased incidence of yeast infections

* Possible role in darkening of the skin (hyperpigmentation) (the area around the nipples and the face are some of the areas particularly prone to this effect)

Progestin

(These effects are seen both with combination birth control pills and progestin-only methods.)

* Irregular bleeding (most common side effect)

* Unexpected flow of breast milk

* Abdominal pain or cramps, diarrhea, nausea

* Fatigue, tiredness, weakness, trouble sleeping

* Hot flashes, decreased sex drive, irritability, or other mood changes

* Acne or skin rash

* Weight gain

* Swelling of the face, ankles, or feet

* Gum disease (periodontal disease) (certain progestins, such as desogestrel, increase the risk for gum disease, while others do not; it's not known why only some progestins affect this risk)

When estrogen and progestin are used together, like in the combination pill, their overall effect can be quite different from the individual side effects. For instance, both estrogen and progestin affect a woman's naturally occurring testosterone levels. Estrogen tends to decrease the testosterone, while progestin tends to increase it. However, the net effect is an almost 5 percent decrease in free testosterone. This decrease means the combination pill reduces testosterone-related side effects, such as acne and hirsutism.

The Pill's most common side effects fall in the nuisance category— for example, breakthrough bleeding. However, Pill hormones, just like natural hormones, have the potential to cause serious side effects. Although these effects are quite rare, if you're considering using the Pill you should be aware of them so you can recognize warning signs and weigh your risks and benefits when making health decisions.

Some of the warning signs of these serious problems include severe abdominal pain, chest pain, unusual headaches, visual disturbances, or severe pain or swelling in the legs. Following is a more detailed listing of these side effects.

Blood clots and complications:
Deep-vein blood clots (thromboses) form in the leg where they can block blood flow. These clots can also travel to the lungs, where they can cause serious complications or even death. The medical name for this serious condition is venous thromboembolism (VTE). Less often, blood clots can form in the blood vessels of the eye. This can lead to impaired vision, double vision, and even blindness. If you use the Pill, this is how it affects your risk of developing a blood clot problem:

* *Three- to fourfold increased risk in current users (but not in past users).* All women who use the Pill have a small, but increased, risk of developing blood clots. If you don't use the Pill your risk of developing these problems is extremely low: about 1 per 10,000 women per year (i.e., over the course of one year, one woman out of 10,000 is at risk). If you do use it, your risk is still very low, at 1–3 per 10,000 women-years. If you are pregnant, you have the highest risk of all: 5.7 per 10,000 women-years. This risk for Pill users is highest in the first few months after you start taking it. The risk increases with:

• Age
• History of inherited blood clotting defects (thrombophilias)
• Obesity
• Smoking
• Having delivered a baby within the past two to three weeks
• A sedentary lifestyle
• Prolonged bed rest (due to recent surgery, injury, or illness)
• High blood pressure (hypertension)
• High blood sugar (diabetes)

If you have a family history of venous blood clots you should be screened for clotting disorders prior to starting combination pills.

* A possible additional one-and-a-half-to-twofold increased VTE risk if you use some third-generation progestins. Some studies found that women using a Pill brand containing the progestin desogestrel or gestodene had an additional up to twofold increase VTE risk (when compared to women who used a brand containing the progestin levonorgestrel). However, follow-up studies did not confirm this increased risk. Although the clinical relevance of these findings isn't clear, a smart strategy would be to use these progestin brands only if you have a low risk for VTE, you cannot tolerate other brands, or you've made an informed choice.

Stroke:

A stroke is caused by a blockage or rupture of a blood vessel in the brain. It can cause serious disability, like paralysis, or even death. This is what happens to your stroke risk if you use the Pill:

* No increased risk (in certain groups of women only). You don't have an increased risk if you are a healthy nonsmoker and you use a low-dose estrogen brand. However, you are at increased risk if you use a high-dose estrogen brand (more than 50 micrograms).

* Increased risk (in certain groups of women). If you smoke or have migraine headaches or high blood pressure, you have a considerably increased risk, regardless of what pill brand you use.

Heart attack (myocardial infarction):

Blockage of blood vessels in the heart can cause a heart attack, a potentially deadly condition. If you use the Pill, this is what happens to your risk of a heart attack:

* No increased risk with low-dose brands (in certain groups of women only). Regardless of age, if you're a healthy nonsmoker and use a low-dose estrogen pill brand, there's no increased risk for heart attack.

* *Increased risk (in certain groups of women).* If you are over 35 years old and a heavy smoker (more than fifteen cigarettes per day) you have an increased risk. You should not use combination pills at all.

In addition, women in the following groups appear to have an increased risk:

* Smokers taking brands containing a second-generation progestin (levonorgestrel)

* Women with high blood pressure (hypertension) and/or high cholesterol (hyperlipidemia)

Clearly, stroke and heart attack are serious complications of using combination pills. However, the risk they pose, overall, is very low—far lower than the risk of these side effects in a pregnant woman. If you are pregnant you have a twofold higher risk of these complications than if you were taking the Pill.

High blood pressure (hypertension):
Over time, high blood pressure (hypertension) can be dangerous to your health. This is because hypertension can cause blood vessel damage. Unfortunately, in the vast majority of people who develop this problem, the cause is unknown.

* *The Pill increases blood pressure.* The increase is usually by about 8 mm Hg systolic and 6 mm Hg diastolic (mm Hg or millimeter of mercury is the unit of measure used for blood pressure). This doesn't mean you become hypertensive; it means you have a higher pressure than before using the Pill. It appears that both the estrogen and the progestin contribute to this increase. The good news is that the higher blood pressure usually disappears once the pills are stopped and there's no long-term damage. The bad news is that it's not possible to predict in advance who will develop this while using combination pills.

Of course if you already have a history of abnormally high blood pressure, you need to be cautious when using the Pill. For example, if you developed high blood pressure during a pregnancy, use combination pills with caution.

Migraine headaches:
Period-related migraines or headaches occur two days before or after the period, or, for Pill users, during the pill-free (placebo) interval and are due to hormonal fluctuations, in particular estrogen. Migraines with auras are caused by other problems.

> * *If you have migraine headaches their frequency and intensity may become worse while you use the Pill for birth control.* For example, in one study 70 percent of the Pill users reported headaches during the placebo interval. Unfortunately, it's not really possible to predict before you use the Pill what the effect will be in your particular case. Some migraines actually improve.

If you have migraine headaches with auras you should not use the combination pill. It's likely that even a history of this type of migraine headache is associated with an increased risk of stroke. So, if you suffer from migraines with aura, you should not use combination pills at all.

Breast cancer:
> * *The latest data indicates that using the Pill does not increase a woman's risk of developing breast cancer.* (For a detailed discussion, please see chapter 3.)

Cervical cancer:
> * *There's a possible link between the Pill and cervical cancer* (in certain groups of women only). Cervical cancer refers to cancer of the cervix area of the uterus. In women infected with HPV who use the Pill for more than five years, there's an increased

risk of cervical cancer. (See chapter 3.) The nature of the association between the increased risk and Pill use is unclear, and research is under way to resolve this issue. What's unclear is if the increased risk is caused by the pills or by other factors. Here's how these factors might play a role:

Women who use the Pill are less likely to use barrier birth control methods that protect against sexually transmitted infections (STIs), such as the virus that causes genital warts, or human papilloma virus (HPV). Some HPV strains have been linked with cervical cancer. It's not the Pill itself that increases the risk of cervical cancer; rather, not using barrier methods increases the risk. Additionally, women who use the Pill are more likely to visit a doctor and undergo cervical screening. Cervical screening detects cervical cancer. So, if you use the Pill you have a higher chance of having a cervical cancer detected.

Liver cancer:
* *There's no increased risk of liver cancer.* An older study reported an association between long-term (over eight years) Pill use and liver cancer; however, more recent studies support the current view that there's no increased risk. There is a possible link to the development of liver nodules. A liver nodule, mostly noncancerous (benign), is an unusual condition, and the use of the newer, low-dose estrogen brands appears to have reduced this side effect.

Liver and gallbladder disease:
* *There is no additional risk for developing gallbladder disease.* However, gallbladder disease may develop more rapidly in susceptible women. For example, if you already have gallstones, combination pills may worsen the condition.

If you have a history of active liver disease, such as hepatitis, you shouldn't use the Pill. Jaundice is an uncommon side effect of the Pill and the problem clears up when you stop taking it.

Metabolic effects:

Metabolic effects are the effects the Pill has on blood levels of cholesterol, fat, and sugar. Both hormones in the Pill affect these levels—often in opposite ways. For example, estrogen lowers the "bad" cholesterol level, while some progestins raise it. If your cholesterol level is already higher than normal but controlled, it's best to use a pill brand that has desogestrel or norgestimate.

* *The Pill increases triglyceride levels.* For most women with normal levels, this is not significant. However, if you have high triglyceride levels you shouldn't use the Pill.

* *There is no increased risk of developing diabetes mellitus.* If you don't have any blood sugar problems, using the Pill doesn't increase your risk of developing them. If you already suffer from diabetes, using the Pill doesn't worsen it. Women with a history of gestational diabetes should use a low-dose pill brand. (Gestational diabetes is a type of diabetes that develops during pregnancy only.)

Breastfeeding:

* *If you are breastfeeding you shouldn't use the combination pill because the combination pill reduces the amount of breast milk.* Instead, use the progestin-only pill. (We'll discuss this pill in chapter 6.)

Weight:

* *Taking the Pill doesn't cause weight gain* (and newer brands do not cause weight loss). Of course, this doesn't mean that some women who use the Pill don't gain or lose weight—they do. But so do women who don't use the Pill. Bottom line: the effects of the Pill on body weight are small and generally transient.

Finally, it's important to remember that the Pill doesn't offer you any protection from sexually transmitted infections, including human immunodeficiency virus (HIV), the virus that causes acquired immunodeficiency syndrome (AIDS).

Types of Combination Birth Control Pills

Before we see how the Pill is used to manage your period, let's take a look at the types of pills available. (If you're a current Pill user, take a look at your pill pack and follow along to see where your brand fits in.)

Most combination birth control pill brands come in 21- or 28-day packs. Each pill in the 21-day pack is "active," meaning each contains estrogen and progestin. In the 28-day pack, there are seven additional pills—the "inactive" pills. These pills don't have any hormones and are called placebo, or "sugar," pills. They are a different color than the active pills and you take them as a "reminder," so you don't forget your daily pill-taking routine. This comes in handy when you use them for birth control.

One of the newer brands, Mircette, has twenty-one days of active pills, followed by two days of placebo pills and five days of active, estrogen-only pills. Another brand, Minesse, reduces the placebo interval from seven to four days.

Based on the amount of hormones in the active pills, there are three types of pill cycles: monophasic, biphasic, and triphasic. (In general, to manage your period you should use only the monophasic brands.) Let's quickly describe all three types of cycles so you understand the differences.

MONOPHASIC (ONE-PHASE) CYCLE

All active pills in the cycle have the same strength.

A 21-day pack has pills that are all one strength and one color for twenty-one days.

A 28-day pack adds seven placebo pills of a different color.

BIPHASIC (TWO-PHASE) CYCLE

For most brands, all the pills in the cycle have the same amount of estrogen, but two strengths of progestin, which is increased during the second half of the cycle.

A 21-day pack has pills of one strength and color taken for seven or ten days, then a second pill with a different strength and color for the remainder of the cycle.

A 28-day pack has an extra seven placebo pills of a third color.

Several brands contain sequential pills: just estrogen for seven days, then estrogen and progestin for fifteen days (for a 22-day cycle), followed by six pill-free days.

TRIPHASIC (THREE-PHASE) CYCLE

There are three phases in this cycle, with either the same varying amounts of estrogen and varying amounts of progestin. The estrogen dose is higher in the middle of the cycle; progestin usually increases in three steps during the cycle. The duration of each phase and the estrogen/progestin strengths depend on the brand used.

A 21-day pack has pills with three different colors and strengths. First, pills of one strength and color are taken for five to seven days. Then pills of a different strength and color are taken for the next five to seven days. Finally, a third strength and color pill is taken for the reminder of the cycle.

A 28-day pack has an extra seven placebo pills of a fourth color.

How Do You Use Combination Birth Control Pills?

THE BIRTH CONTROL REGIMEN

When you use the Pill for birth control you take a pill once a day, ideally at the same time each day, until the pack is used up. For the 21-day pack, there are seven pill-free days before you start a new pack. There are no pill-free days with the 28-day pack; instead the last seven days are placebo-pill days. Often, the birth control regimen is referred to as the "regular," the "28-day," or the "21/7" monthly regimen (twenty-one days on active pills, seven days off active pills).

Regardless of what brand of combination pill they use, most women experience a monthly fake period (an episode of bleeding). Usually, if you use the 21-day pack, the bleeding occurs at the end of the pack, during the seven pill-free days. If you use the 28-day pack, the bleeding occurs during the seven placebo-pill days.

When you first start using the Pill, you'll begin either on the first

Sunday after your menstrual period starts (the "Sunday start") or during the first twenty-four hours of the period (the "Day 1 start"). These are the most commonly used starts. There's also a "quick-start": you take the first pill on whatever day of the monthly cycle you happen to have your doctor's appointment; and an "immediate start" (like right after a pregnancy termination). Your doctor can go over the details and which start is best for you.

The one thing you have to keep in mind is that, except for a Day 1 start, in general, you need to use a backup method of birth control, like a barrier method, during the first week of taking the Pill. (That's because it takes about one week for the hormones in the Pill to offer you full pregnancy protection.)

✳ NOTE

If you are sexually active, it's always a good idea to keep a backup method of birth control handy, just in case. Condoms, the sponge (Pharmatex,* Protectaid,* Today*) or the Ovès* cap are all good options— they're easy to use and are available over the counter.

*not yet available in the United States.

Bottom line: *When you use the Pill for birth control, you no longer have a menstrual period.* This is normal, and it's the way the Pill works. (See chapters 2 and 4 for more detail.) What you do have is a monthly fake period—a made-up bleeding event, which we discussed at length in chapter 4.

THE MENSTRUAL MANAGEMENT REGIMEN

Now that we've reviewed the birth control pill regimen, it's easy to understand why the combination pill is a commonly used method of active menstrual management. When you use the Pill, you don't have a menstrual period for the duration of use. So right off the bat, you have the power to control whether you have a period. Use the Pill and you stop having periods; discontinue the Pill and your period returns. Furthermore, when you use the Pill you have a fake period, whose frequency you can control. You can decide to have no fake periods or fewer fake periods. It's up to you. Your decision will determine your regimen options.

For most women the goals of using menstrual management can be divided into four basic ones:

* Regulating the period

* Reducing the menstrual bleeding and/or other period-related problems

* Decreasing the number of periods

* Stopping having periods and/or fake periods altogether for a while

Of course, the underlying reasons why you'd want to achieve any of these goals vary and are unique to you. For the moment, it doesn't matter why you'd choose to use period control, but rather what you're trying to achieve. So, based on your end goal, the period control pill regimens you can use fall into two broad groups: minimal control and full control.

Minimal period control regimen:
If you want only to regulate your periods, decrease the blood flow, or reduce the pain and cramps, you can start using combination birth control pills on the regular, on/off schedule.

Think of this minimal degree of period control as tweaking your period. Minimal control works best if your end goal is to:

* Regulate the period

* Reduce menstrual bleeding and/or other period-related problems

For example, this regimen will help if:

* You have irregular cycles and you want to know when your bleeding will start.

* Your flow is a bit heavy and you would like to have a lighter flow.

* Your period lasts for five or seven days and you'd like to have it last for two to four days.

* Occasionally you have bothersome menstrual cramps that you would prefer to avoid.

The regular birth control pill regimen can help you achieve any of these changes. The way you take the Pill is the same as if you were using it for pregnancy protection—in a cyclical, 21/7, on/off way. One important reminder: just because you're using the same regimen doesn't mean you *have* to be sexually active. Remember, *there's no sexual activity requirement built into using the Pill for menstrual management.*

For this type of regimen, you can use any pill brand except Seasonale. You can use any type—mono-, bi-, or triphasic—if you're using them only for minor cycle control. (See the Appendix for a listing of available combination pill brands.)

Regardless of what brand you use, you will be taking an active pill for twenty-one days followed by seven days of no pills or a placebo, during which time you will get a fake period. In contrast to your natural period, the Pill-induced period will come on a regular schedule—when you stop taking the (active) pills—and it will last fewer days, the flow will be lighter, and there will be less, if any, cramping or discomfort.

Using this regimen can sometimes also help women who have more serious period-related problems. For example, let's say you suffer from very heavy bleeding, anemia, or endometriosis. This cyclical regimen can be a first step: you try it first to see if it does the trick. If it does, great! If not, you can always switch to the full control regimen.

Another group of women who can benefit from first using this regimen is women who've never used the Pill before. Because it takes your body time to adjust to the Pill, the highest frequency of nuisance side effects, like breakthrough bleeding or spotting, is during the first two to three months of use. You're also more likely to have spotting during the first few months of a full-control regimen, compared to the minimal-control regimen. So, if you've never used the Pill, in order to minimize your chance of spotting, start with the on/off regimen for two to three months, and then switch to the continuous one (discussed in the next section).

As for how often and how long you use this regimen, it depends on your particular circumstances. You can use this minimal-control regimen once in a while, for example only during the summer. The same applies to how long you use it. You can use it short-term, let's say for five months while you're taking a semester abroad, or for years at a time, say while in graduate school. (One note of caution: once you stop using the regimen, whatever period-related problems you had before will most likely return.)

If you don't want to (or shouldn't) have a monthly fake period, the minimal-control pill regimen is not for you. You need to use the full-control regimen.

Full period control regimen:
The time to use the full period control regimen is when your goals are to:

* Decrease the number of periods

* Stop having periods and/or fake periods altogether for a while

With full period control you decide when the bleeding starts and how many fake periods you have. Here are some examples of situations where this pill regimen may be the best choice:

* You don't want to have a period every month.

* You're already using the Pill for birth control but suffer from fake period–related problems.

* Your health will benefit from not having a monthly episode of bleeding for an extended period of time.

When you use any of the full-control regimens, you take the Pill continuously—there are no off weeks. In other words, you take a pill once a day, ideally at the same time each day, until you want to have a fake period. At that time, you stop taking pills for seven days, during which time you'll have the withdrawal bleeding. Then you start all over again.

You should use either Seasonale or a monophasic pill brand for these regimens. This is because the triphasic brands tend to cause too many minor side effects due to the increased fluctuations in the hormone levels, not to mention the confusion they tend to cause when it comes to which color pill you're supposed to take. (See Appendix A for a listing of monophasic pill brands.) However, if your pill brand is a triphasic one, you should be able to use it; just consult with your doctor.

Just to give you a general idea, there are several full-control continuous regimen possibilities, both variable and fixed.

The idea behind a *variable* regimen is that you take a pill continuously until you spontaneously experience breakthrough bleeding or spotting (BTB or BTS). Then you stop taking the Pill (anywhere from two to seven days off the pills), allow for a fake period, and then restart. This type of regimen gives you less control than the fixed one.

With the *fixed* regimen you take a fixed number of pill packs continuously, followed by two to seven days pill-free, during which time you'll have a fake period. For example, you can take two packs in a row (49-day regimen—forty-two days on, seven days off), or four packs in a row (91-day regimen—eighty-four days on, seven days off), or twelve packs in a row, or any other chosen fixed number of packs. (Your physician can help you decide which number is best for you.)

Since Seasonale, the only brand specifically packaged for continuous use, is a fixed 91-day regimen, let's use the 91-day regimen to illustrate how you take the pills.

For this regimen you take a pill every day for eighty-four days. Then you stop taking pills for seven days to allow for an episode of withdrawal bleeding. Again, this bleeding will be light, short, and pain-free. Also, it doesn't matter if you experience breakthrough bleeding or spotting during the eighty-four days—you continue to take the fixed number of pills.

Here's how the 91-day regimen works if you're using three different pill brands: the new pill Seasonale, a 21-day pill pack brand, or a 28-day pill pack brand:

If you use Seasonale, take one pink pill for eighty-four days, preferably at the same time each day. Once the pink pills are finished, take the seven white pills. These are the placebo pills, and this is when you'll have the fake period.

If you use a 21-day pack, take one pill each day, preferably at the same time each day. Once the pack is finished, instead of waiting for seven days to start another pack, start a new pack right away. Do this for four packs (eighty-four days) in a row. After the fourth pack, take one week off—no pills for seven days. You'll most likely have a fake period during this time. After the seven days, start the sequence again.

If you use a 28-day pack, you take one pill each day for twenty-one days in a row, preferably at the same time each day. Because you'll be using a monophasic brand, all the twenty-one pills you take will be the same color. Once you finish all the same-color twenty-one pills, discard the pack. (There should be seven pills left in the pack; these are the placebo, or inert, pills. These pills will also be of one color, which will be different from the color of the other twenty-one pills.) Start a new pack right away and repeat the regimen—take twenty-one pills, throw out the remaining seven. Do this for four packs (eighty-four days) in a row. After the fourth pack, take one week off—no pills for seven days. You'll most likely have a fake period during this time. After the seven days, start the sequence again.

For all the brand types—Seasonale, a 21-day pack brand, and a 28-day pack brand—the most common pill-free interval is seven days. However, that's not written in stone. You can shorten this interval to, for example, four days. For Seasonale, take only four white pills, then discard the rest and start a new Seasonale pack. For the 21- or 28-day pill pack, instead of waiting for seven days to start a new pack, you start it after four days. Shortening the pill-free interval can give you several advantages. The fake period is shorter and there's less blood lost. Also, if you suffer from fake period–related problems, or your health is made worse by bleeding, the shorter the interval the better. One note of caution: don't take more than seven days off! There's an increased chance of spotting and you may become pregnant if you're sexually active.

Of course, the 91-day regimen (with four fake periods a year) described above is just one of the fixed-regimen options. Other regimens that have been studied are the 42-day regimen (with a fake period every other month), and the 168-day regimen (with two fake periods per year), and the 336-day one (with a fake period once a year); and many other regimens have been used in clinical practice. However, the only FDA-approved regimen is the 91-day one. Bottom line: your health-care professional is in the best position to advise which regimen and which pill brand would benefit you most.

If you're wondering why the 91-day regimen was selected by the FDA, the answer is simple: surveys and polls have found that the preferred frequency of bleeding for most women is every three months, so that was the regimen submitted for approval. Much like the frequency of the monthly fake period, which was determined by social, political, and religious factors, the frequency of the fake period for the 91-day regimen is not driven by medical reasons. The bottom line: consult with your physician about the fixed regimen that will best fit your particular circumstances.

No matter which regimen you're using, the hormone levels from the Pill don't build up, regardless of how long you take the pills continuously, and fertility doesn't appear to be affected. It takes the body about twenty-four hours to eliminate the hormones in one pill, regardless if you've been taking the Pill for one week or one year. Moreover, even if you're using one of the continuous regimens in which the total dose of hormones is higher because you're taking the Pill without a break for more days (when compared to the regular birth control regimen), the hormones don't build up in your system. (For more on this, see chapter 4.)

Just as with the minimal-control regimen, you can use the full-control regimen only occasionally—for a special event—or frequently. Also, you can use it for a short period of time or long-term. If you plan to use period control for a short time—for a one-time event like a honeymoon—it's best if you plan in advance. In other words, to minimize your chances of spotting, start a fixed, full-control regimen about three months before the planned event.

About Specific Brands of Combination Pills

Dozens of products are available, with different levels of hormones and designed for one, two, or three phases. See Appendix A for a complete list.

SEASONALE

Seasonale is a combination pill brand that, at the time of this writing, is the only one approved by the FDA expressly to carry a continuous use dosage on label. Each active (pink) pill has estrogen (0.03 mg ethinyl estradiol) and progestin (0.15 mg levonorgestrel). The seven placebo pills are white. Because this brand is specifically packaged for continuous use, one pack has a total of ninety-one pills (eighty-four pink active pills and seven white placebo pills), arranged in three trays of twenty-eight pills each. The last tray contains the placebo pills.

Because Seasonale is currently the only FDA-approved brand packaged for menstrual management, if you've never used the Pill before, or if you're concerned that you might not properly remember how to follow your doctor's instructions for the brand you're currently using, this is the most convenient brand for you to use.

(*Note: despite the fact that Seasonale is the only FDA-approved brand for continuous use, you doctor is in the best position to advise which brand you should use.)

Resource: http://seasonale.com/default.sap (site maintained by the manufacturer).

On the Horizon

Yasmin, a low-dose monophasic pill brand containing a newer type of progestin (drospirenone), could soon be available in a menstrual management package. Women who used this brand continuously for up to four and a half months experienced significantly less breast tenderness and an improvement in period-related pain. Other continuous brands under development are DP3 and SeasonaleLo, a lower dose version of Seasonale.

The Skin Patch (Ortho Evra)

The birth control skin patch is a small, smooth square measuring 1¾ inches on each of its four sides. The patch has three layers—an outer protective one, a middle adhesive one, and a clear release liner that you remove just prior to applying the patch. (The hormones are in the middle layer.) The patch has two hormones—a combination of 0.75 milligrams of estrogen (ethinyl estradiol) and 6.0 milligrams of progestin (norelgestromin). It requires a prescription and an initial office visit to a physician. Subsequent patches are self-applied. The brand name for the birth control patch is Ortho Evra and it was approved for use in the United States in 2001. The patch is already available in Latin America (Mexico, Argentina, Brazil, and Columbia), Canada, Ireland and the United Kingdom, Germany, and Finland. There are plans to introduce it in more countries.

Who Can Use the Skin Patch?

Anyone who can use combination birth control pills can use the skin patch. (See the list of cautionary factors on pages 139–140.)

Who Cannot Use the Skin Patch?

Anyone who can't use combination birth control pills should not use the skin patch. (See pages 140–141 for a detailed list.)

In addition, if you weigh more than 198 pounds (90 kg) use the skin patch with caution. (The pregnancy protection efficacy of the patch may be decreased with increased body weight.)

Advantages of Using the Skin Patch

* *It can be used for birth control.*

* *You may be able to use it to control your menstrual period.*

* *You don't have to remember to take a pill every day.*

* *It may offer you additional health benefits.*

Theoretically, the skin patch offers you the same non-birth-control-related health benefits as birth control pills. However, because this is a new method, more long-term studies are needed to confirm this.

Disadvantages of Using the Skin Patch

The same general side effects associated with any combination hormonal birth control method are associated with using the skin patch. (See pages 145–152 for a full list). Because smoking independently increases the risk of serious heart and blood vessel problems, if you use the skin patch you should strongly consider not smoking at all. Also, this method offers you no protection from sexually transmitted infections like HIV/AIDS.

The particular disadvantages associated with using the skin patch are these:

* *The skin patch does not stick in about 5 percent of women.*

* *The patch can become partially or completely detached.*

* *You may forget to change your patch.*

* *You may experience an allergic reaction or skin irritation at the application site.* If the skin where you applied the patch be-

comes irritated you can remove and discard the patch and apply a new one, immediately, to a different area. You keep this new patch on only until the usual "patch change day." (See below for an explanation of the "patch change day.")

* *You may have more breast discomfort and breakthrough bleeding and/or spotting.* More women who use the skin patch experience these side effects during the first one to two months of use, when compared to Pill users. However, by the third month of use, patch and Pill users have similar rates.

* *It is less effective in women who weigh more than 198 pounds (90 kg).*

How Do You Use the Skin Patch?

The patch releases a steady daily dose of each hormone: 20 micrograms of ethinyl estradiol and 150 micrograms of norelgestromin. The hormones pass through the skin into the bloodstream. This is called the transdermal route. Once in the bloodstream, the hormones are carried to their target organs. One patch has enough hormones to last for about nine days.

You apply the skin patch yourself, on the skin of the upper outer arm, abdomen, upper torso (front and back, excluding the breasts), or buttocks.

To remove the patch, you simply peel it off and throw it away. The patch is disposable and the same patch is not meant to be reused.

THE BIRTH CONTROL REGIMEN

When you use the skin patch for birth control, the patch is applied and removed in a cyclical, on/off way. In other words, you apply the patch and leave it on for seven days in a row. Then you remove it at the beginning of the second week, throw it out, and apply a new patch immediately. (Choose a different skin location for the new patch, to avoid irritating the skin.) You leave the new patch on for another week. After three weeks, and three patches, the fourth week is patch-free. During this patch-free week you'll have the fake period.

The first time you use the skin patch, you can use either a "Day 1" or a "Sunday" start. For a Day 1 start you apply the first patch on the first day of menstruation. For a Sunday start you apply it on the first Sunday after your period starts.

A Sunday start regimen requires you use a backup birth control method for the first seven days. This allows the hormones in the skin patch to give you full pregnancy protection. Any barrier method, like the condom, the Ovès cap, or the sponge, is a good option. The exception to using the backup birth control method is if you chose a Sunday start and your menstrual period happens to start that Sunday. In that case you apply the first patch that Sunday and you don't need a backup method.

Once you start using the patch, every week you should apply every new patch on the same day of the week. For example, let's say that the first time you ever used the skin patch you chose a Day 1 start, and that your period happened to start on a Tuesday. So, you apply the first patch on Tuesday, and this day now becomes the "patch change day." Any subsequent patch changes should be done on a Tuesday.

THE MENSTRUAL MANAGEMENT REGIMEN

Theoretically, you could use the skin patch for menstrual management, by applying and removing the patch in a continuous way. In other words, you'd wear a patch for seven days in a row and then you'd replace it with a new one right away, at a different body location. You'd continue to do this for two to three months in a row, until you decided to have a bleeding episode. At that time you wouldn't use a patch for one week, during which time you'd have a fake period. Once the week is over, you'd resume the continuous regimen.

Because the skin patch is a relatively new method, the continuous regimen hasn't been extensively studied. The results of a study that looked at women using the patch for three months continually for one year should be available soon.

What to Do if the Skin Patch Becomes Partially or Completely Detached

Occasionally, the patch may become partially or completely detached accidentally. What you do if this happens depends on why you're using the patch and how long it's been detached.

If the patch detaches and you notice it before twenty-four hours have passed, simply try to reapply it to the same spot, or immediately replace it with a new patch. If you use the patch for pregnancy protection, you don't need to use a backup birth control method. Your "patch change day" remains the same and you continue to use the cyclical regimen. If you're using the patch to control your period, you should also be fine. Just reapply the patch if possible (or apply a new one) and keep using the continuous regimen.

If more than twenty-four hours have passed before you notice that the patch has detached, you must apply a new patch to take its place. If you're using the patch for birth control, this now becomes the new "patch change day." You will need to use a backup method, like a barrier method, for the next seven days. If you're using the patch to control your period, just replace it by applying a new patch and carry on with the continuous regimen. Be aware that you might notice some spotting for a few days.

Resource: www.orthoevra.com (site maintained by the manufacturer).

On the Horizon

Schering AG is developing a new birth control patch that will have a low-dose estrogen (ethinyl estradiol) and progestin (gestodene). The advantages of this patch: a smaller size and a superior appearance (it's transparent). Submission for regulatory approval is planned for some time later this year.

The Vaginal Ring (NuvaRing)

The birth control vaginal ring is a soft, thin, flexible plastic ring. It contains a combination of estrogen and progestin: 2.7 milligrams ethinyl estradiol and 11.7 milligrams etonogestrel. The ring requires a doctor's prescription and an initial physician office visit. Subsequent vaginal rings are self-applied at home. The brand name for the vaginal ring is NuvaRing. It was launched in 2001 and became available in the United States and worldwide after mid 2002.

Who Can Use the Vaginal Ring?

Anyone who can use combination birth control pills can use the vaginal ring. (See the list of cautionary factors on pages 139–140.)

Who Cannot Use the Vaginal Ring?

Anyone who can't use combination birth control pills should not use the vaginal ring. (See pages 140–141 for a detailed list.)

In addition, if you have any of the following conditions, you shouldn't use the vaginal ring:

* **Active lesions on or infections of the vagina or cervix.** You should wait until these problems are treated before using the ring.

* **Any condition that may distort the anatomy of the vagina.** You should use the ring with caution if you have a dropped (prolapsed) uterus, bladder, or rectum. Any of these conditions can make insertion or removal of the ring difficult.

Advantages of Using the Vaginal Ring

* *It can be used for birth control.*

* *You can use it to manage your menstrual period.*

* *You don't have to remember to take a pill every day or change a skin patch once a week.*

* *It may offer you additional health benefits.*

Theoretically, the ring offers you the same non-birth-control-related health benefits as birth control pills. However, because this is a new method, more long-term studies are needed to confirm this.

Disadvantages of Using the Vaginal Ring

The same general side effects associated with any combination hormonal birth control method are associated with using the vaginal ring. (See pages 145–152 for a full list). Because smoking increases the risk of serious heart and blood vessel disease, if you use the vaginal ring you should strongly consider not smoking. Also, the vaginal ring offers no protection from sexually transmitted infections like HIV/AIDS.

The particular disadvantages associated with using the vaginal ring are these:

* *Vaginal irritation, discharge, and infections (most common).*

* *Headaches.*

* *The ring may become dislodged or slip out from the vagina.*

* *Foreign-body sensation.* Some women may feel the ring inside the vagina at times. To try to correct this problem, reposition the ring: take the ring out and immediately reinsert it. Also, if you or your partner feels the ring while having sex, you can take the ring out and reinsert it once you're done. Make sure, however, that you don't leave the ring out for more than three hours.

How Do You Use the Vaginal Ring?

The ring releases a small, steady daily amount of each hormone in the vagina every day: 15 micrograms of ethinyl estradiol and 120 micrograms of etonogestrel. The hormones pass through the lining of the vagina into the bloodstream. This is called the *transvaginal* route. Once in the bloodstream, the hormones are carried to their target organs. One ring has enough hormones to last for approximately thirty-five days.

You insert the ring into the vagina by holding it between two fingers, pressing the edges together, and pushing it in as you would a tampon. The ring doesn't need to fit exactly over the cervix because it's not a barrier method.

To remove the ring, you either hook the index finger under the forward rim or hold the rim between two fingers and pull it out. If you remove the ring temporarily during sexual intercourse (remember: for no more than three hours) you can reinsert it. However, once you remove a ring at the end of its useful life, you throw it out. The vaginal ring is disposable and is not meant to be reused.

THE BIRTH CONTROL REGIMEN

When you use the vaginal ring for pregnancy protection, you insert and remove the ring in a cyclical way. In other words, you insert the ring into the vagina and leave it in for three weeks (twenty-one days) in a row. At the beginning of the fourth week, you remove it and throw it out. Then, you don't use a ring at all for the fourth week. This is when the fake period will usually occur. After this ring-free week, you insert a new ring and start all over again.

The first time you use the ring you can insert it on any day from Day 1 (the first day of menstrual bleeding) to Day 5 of your menstrual cycle. It doesn't matter if you still have your period. You need to use a backup birth control method, like a barrier method, for the first seven days to allow time for the ring's hormones to start working and protect you from a pregnancy. You can use any barrier method except the diaphragm or any modified diaphragm device, like a Lea's shield, FemCap, or Vimule or Dumas cap. This is because the ring may interfere with positioning these devices correctly into the vagina.

THE MENSTRUAL MANAGEMENT REGIMEN

To control your menstrual period, you use the ring in a continuous way. In other words, you insert the ring into the vagina and leave it in for either three or four weeks (twenty-eight days). After that, you remove it and throw it out. Then you replace the old ring, immediately, with a new one. There is no ring-free week between the old and the new ring. You continue to do this for two to possibly three or more months (see below). At the end of that interval you stop using the ring for seven days. You'll have the fake period during these seven ring-free days.

You can use the vaginal ring this way because it has enough hormones to last for approximately thirty-five days. However, because the ring is a relatively new method, the continuous regimen hasn't been extensively studied. For example, using the ring continuously for two months doesn't cause unfavorable changes in the vagina. Using it for longer intervals might. In an ongoing extended-wear study, women have been using the vaginal ring (replacing it every three weeks) continuously for six weeks, twelve weeks, and twelve months. Preliminary results should be available in late 2004.

What to Do if the Ring Slips Out or Is Removed Accidentally

For both the birth control regimen as well as for the menstrual management regimen, you can remove the ring during sexual intercourse (but for no more than three hours). However, occasionally, the ring may slip out of the vagina accidentally. As soon as you notice this, reinsert it into the vagina. What you do after that depends on what you're using the ring for and on how long it's been out of the vagina.

If the ring has been outside the vagina for less than three hours, and you're using the ring for pregnancy protection, you don't need to use a backup birth control method. Just reinsert the ring and continue the usual cyclical birth control schedule. If this occurs while you're using the ring for menstrual management, you should be fine. Reinsert the ring and carry on with the continuous-use regimen.

If the ring has been out of the vagina for more than three hours, and you're using it for pregnancy protection, reinsert it and use a backup method, like condoms, for seven days. If you're using the ring for period control, reinsert it and carry on, but be aware that you might experience some spotting for a few days.

Resource: www.nuvaring.com (site maintained by the manufacturer).

On the Horizon

A vaginal ring containing only one hormone, a progestin (nestorone), designed to be used for six continuous months is currently under development. One of the advantages of the ring is that it's very well suited for use by breastfeeding women.

In this chapter we've reviewed the combination pill, the skin patch, and the vaginal ring—the three methods that can be used to actively manage your period. The next chapter is dedicated to discussing the passive menstrual management methods—the progestin-only pill, the shots, implants, and hormone-releasing intrauterine devices (IUDs)—as well as various surgical methods.

Chapter Five Bibliography

Cunningham GF, Gant NF, Leveno KJ, *et al*, eds. Estrogen plus progestin contraceptives. In: *Williams Obstetrics*. 21st ed. New York, NY: McGraw-Hill; 2001:1525.

Davis A, Godwin A, Lippman J, *et al.* Triphasic norgestimate-ethinyl estradiol for treating dysfunctional uterine bleeding. *Obstet Gynecol*. 2000;96:913–20.

Panser LA, Phipps WR. Type of oral contraceptive in relation to acute, initial episode of pelvic inflammatory disease. *Contraception*. 1991;43:91–9.

DeCherney A. Bone-sparing properties of oral contraceptives. *Am J Obstet Gynecol.* 1996;174:15–20.

Pasco JA, Kotowicz MA, Henry MJ, *et al.* Oral contraceptives and bone mineral density: a population based study. *Am J Obstet Gynecol.* 2000;182:265–9.

Michaëlsson K, Baron JA, Farahmand BY, *et al.* Oral contraceptive use and the risk of hip fracture: a case control study. *Lancet.* 1999;353: 1481–4.

(See also chapter 3 for cancer risk.)

Kaiser Family Foundation. National survey on public perceptions about contraception. Market Facts Survey, January 19–21, 1996.

American College of Obstetricians and Gynecologists. The pill at 40: women say it's safer, has extra benefits but not covered by insurance. Gallup Survey, April 7–21, 2000. http://www.acog.org/from_home/publications/press_releases/nr05-02-00-1.cfm. Accessed May 14, 2004.

Adams Hillard PJ. When should you induce amenorrhea? *Contemp Ob/Gyn.* Jun 2003;48(6):60–74.

Stabinsky SA, Einstein M, Breen JL. Modern treatments of menorrhagia attributable to dysfunctional uterine bleeding. *Obst Gynecol Survey.* 1999;54:61–72.

Cunningham GF, Gant NF, Leveno KJ, *et al*, eds. Sterilization. In: *Williams Obstetrics.* 21st ed. New York, NY: McGraw-Hill; 2001: 1556.

Lloyd T, Taylor DS, Lin HM, *et al.* Oral contraceptive use by teenage women does not affect peak bone mass: a longitudinal study. *Fertil Steril.* 2000 Oct;74(4):734–8.

Cromer BA, Blair JM, Mahan JD, *et al.* A prospective comparison of bone density in adolescent girls receiving depot medroxyprogesterone acetate (Depo-Provera), levonorgestrel (Norplant), or oral contraceptives. *J Pediatr.* 1996;129:671–6.

Hatcher RA, Trussel J, Stewart F, *et al. Contraceptive Technology.* 17th rev. ed. New York: Ardent Media; 1998.

Sulak PJ. Should your patient be on extended-use OCs? *Contemp Ob Gyn.* 2003 Sep;48(9):35–46.

Borgelt-Hansen L. Oral contraceptives: an update on health benefits and risks. *J Am Pharm Assoc.* 2001;41(6):875–86.

Rosenberg L, Palmer JR, Zauber AG, *et al*. A case-control study of oral contraceptive use and invasive epithelial ovarian cancer. *Am J Epidemiol*. 1994;139:654–61.

Ness RB, Grisso JA, Klapper J, *et al*, and the SHARE Study Group. Risk of ovarian cancer in relation to estrogen and progestin dose and use characteristics of oral contraceptives. *Am J Epidemiol*. 2000;152:233–41.

Gross TP, Schlesselman JJ. The estimated effect of oral contraceptive use on the cumulative risk of epithelial ovarian cancer. *Obstet Gynecol*. 1994;83:419–24.

Schlesselman JJ. Risk of endometrial cancer in relation to use of combined oral contraceptives: a practitioner's guide to meta-analysis. *Hum Reprod*. 1997;12:1851–63.

Jick SS, Walker AM, Jick H. Oral contraceptives and endometrial cancer. *Obstet Gynecol*. 1993;82:931–5.

(See also chapter 3.)

Stern RS. The prevalence of acne on the basis of physical examination. *J Am Acad Dermatol*. 1992;26:931–5.

Thorneycroft IH, Stanczyk FZ, Bradshaw KD, *et al*. Effects of low-dose oral contraceptives on androgenic markers and acne. *Contraception*. 1999;60(5):255–262.

Panser LA, Phipps WR. Type of oral contraceptive in relation to acute initial episode of pelvic inflammatory disease. *Contraception*. 1991;43: 91–9.

Rosenberg MJ, Waugh MS. Oral contraceptive discontinuation: a prospective evaluation of frequency and reasons. *Am J Obstet Gynecol*. 1998;179:577–82.

Speroff L. Bone mineral density and hormonal contraception. In: *Dialogues in Contraception*. Summer 2002;7(5):1–3, 8.

Breitkopf DM, Rosen MP, Young SL, *et al*. Efficacy of second versus third generation oral contraceptives in the treatment of hirsutism. *Contraception*. 2003 May;67(5):349–53.

Doran MF, Crowson CS, O'Fallon WM, *et al*. The effect of oral contraceptives and estrogen replacement therapy on the risk of RA: a population based study. *J Rheumatol*. 2004 Feb;31(2): 207–13.

Burkman RT. Oral contraceptives: current status. *Clin Obstet Gynecol*. 2001;44:62–72.

Burkman RT, Heinemann. Progestin and thrombosis. In: *Dialogues in Contraception*. Winter 2001;7(3):5–8.

Cunningham GF, Gant NF, Leveno KJ, *et al*, eds. Estrogen plus progestin contraceptives. In: *Williams Obstetrics*. 21st ed. New York, NY: McGraw-Hill; 2001: 1528–9.

Sulak PJ, Scow RD, Preece C, *et al*. Hormone withdrawal symptoms in oral contraceptive users. *Obstet Gynecol*. 2000;95(2):261–6.

(See chapter 3 for breast and cervical cancer.)

Cunningham GF, Gant NF, Leveno KJ, *et al*, eds. Estrogen plus progestin contraceptives. In: *Williams Obstetrics*. 21st ed. New York, NY: McGraw-Hill; 2001: 1526–7.

Burkman RT, Kaunitz AM. Oral contraceptives: newer formulations and new data. Weight changes. In: *Dialogues in Contraception*. Spring 2003;8(1):2–3.

Shortened pill-free interval delivered by new 20 mcg pill. Organon's Mircette scheduled for U.S. debut this summer. *Contracept Technol Update*. 1998 Jul;19(7):85–7.

Wyeth Pharma: Minesse site (in German). http://www.minesse.at/. Accessed May 15, 2004.

Zieman M, Nelson A. Oral contraceptives: choose when—and whether—to bleed. *Female Patient*. 2003 Oct;28(10):41–2.

Burkman RT, Miller L. Extended and continuous use of hormonal contraceptives. In: *Dialogues in Contraception*. Winter 2004;8(4):2.

Komaat H, Geerdink MH, Klitsie JW. The acceptance of a 7-week cycle with a modern low-dose oral contraceptive (Minulet). *Contraception*. 1992 Feb;45(2):119–27.

Cachrimanidou AC, Hellberg D, Nilsson S, *et al*. Long-interval treatment regimen with a desogestrel-containing oral contraceptive. *Contraception*. 1993 Sep;48(3):205–16.

Sulak PJ, Cressman BE, Waldrop E, *et al*. Extending the duration of active oral contraceptive pills to manage hormone withdrawal symptoms. *Obstet Gynecol*. 1997;89:179–183.

Miller L, Notter KM. Menstrual reduction with extended use of combination oral contraceptive pills: randomized controlled trial. *Obstet Gynecol*. 2001 Nov;98(5 Pt 1):771–8

Sulak PJ, Kuehl TJ, Ortiz M, *et al*. Acceptance of altering the standard

21-day/7-day oral contraceptive regimen to delay menses and reduce hormone withdrawal symptoms. *Am J Obstet Gynecol.* 2002;186:1142–9.

Anderson FD. The safety and efficacy of Seasonale, a novel 91-day extended oral contraceptive regimen. *Obstet Gynecol.* 2002;99(Suppl):26S.

Miller L, Hughes JP. Continuous combination oral contraceptive pills to eliminate withdrawal bleeding: a randomized trial. *Obstet Gynecol.* 2003;101:653–661.

Seasonale. Prescribing information. Duramed Pharmaceuticals, Inc. 2003.

Sillem M, Schneider R, Heithecker R, *et al.* Use of an oral contraceptive containing drospirenone in an extended regimen. *Eur J Contracep Reprod Health Care.* 2003;8:162–9.

Ortho Evra product prescribing information. Ortho-McNeil Pharmaceuticals, Inc. May 2003.

Physician Service Department. Women's Healthcare Section. Ortho-McNeil Pharmaceuticals, Inc. Personal communication.

Philip Smits, MD. Schering R&D Day 2003. Berlin, 26 June 2003.

Darney PD. Current trends in contraception-extended-cycle options. Vaginal ring. *Female Patient.* 2003 Dec;28(Suppl):S20–1.

Mishell DR Jr. Vaginal contraceptive rings. *Ann Med* 1993;25:191–197.

Davies GC, Feng LX, Newton JR, *et al.* The effects of a combined contraceptive vaginal ring releasing ethinyloestradiol and 3-keto-desogestrel on vaginal flora. *Contraception* 1992;45:511–518.

Aarts JM, Miller L. Design of an open-label, randomized, multicenter trial of continuous regimens with NuvaRing. *Obstet Gynecol.* 2003;101(45):145.

Massai R, Diaz S, Jackanicz T, Croxatto HB. Vaginal rings for contraception in lactating women. *Steroids.* 2000 Oct–Nov;65(10–11):703–7.

Blanche V, Alvarez-Sanchez F, Faundes A. Progestin-only contraceptive rings. *Steroids.* 2000 Oct–Nov;65(10–11):687–91.

6

All the Rest

Progestin-Only Pills, Shots, Implants, Intrauterine Devices (IUDs), and Surgery

* * *

Mira is a thirty-eight-year-old office manager. She runs a busy, two-pediatrician practice and she loves the fast pace, the children, and the job satisfaction. However, now, between her many responsibilities, the constant need to keep the doctors on schedule, and her heavy periods, Mira has decided she's had enough. Her periods have always been regular, but heavy and prolonged. She put up with it through college, while raising two children, and while playing an active, leadership role in her church and community. Now Mira has decided to use menstrual management. Because she smokes, Mira isn't comfortable using a period control method with estrogen. Although she would prefer not to have any bleeding at all, she decides she wouldn't mind if she still had some monthly bleeding, as long as the flow was lighter and lasted only a few days.

Just like Mira, some women interested in menstrual management either don't want to or can't use a hormonal method of birth control that has estrogen. So what should they do? Is there a way for these women to take advantage of the benefits offered by period control? Yes, there is. For these women, passive menstrual management provides several solutions.

In the previous chapter we mentioned that the combination hormonal methods allow you to decide whether you have a menstrual period or not: once you start using any of the methods, you no longer have a menstrual period. However, you do have a monthly fake period. With active management you control whether you have a fake period, how often, and, more or less, how long and how heavy the bleeding. Passive menstrual management gives you less control. However, it does allow you to:

* Have shorter and lighter bleeding, consequently reducing several common period-related problems

* Bleed less frequently

* Not bleed at all for a while

What you don't have with this type of menstrual management is control over whether or not you have a period, and the frequency of bleeding. For example, many women stop having both fake and real periods when they use any one of the passive management methods. The problem is it's not possible to predict which women will experience this effect. Nor do you have a way to regulate the bleeding. You'll most likely bleed less frequently than if you weren't using any type of menstrual management, but you'll also most likely bleed at irregular intervals. (More on that later.) Clearly, passive period control is best suited for women who can't or don't want to use the active management methods.

The methods used for passive period control are:

* Progestin-only birth control pill

* Shots

* Implants

* Hormone-releasing intrauterine device (IUD)

Although all these methods are dual use—you can use them for both birth control and period control—in our discussion, we'll only concentrate on the characteristics that relate to menstrual management.

Progestin-Only Pills

The progestin-only pill (POP) has only one hormone: a progestin. This progestin is a man-made version of the natural hormone progesterone made by the body. There are two types of POPs:

* Mini-dose POPs (the "mini" pill)
* Full-dose POPs (the "macropill")

These type of pills have been around for decades, although they are less popular than their two-hormone counterpart, the combination pill. There are numerous brands of POPs, they require a prescription, and they are available worldwide. Some of the newer mini-dose POP brands and the full-dose POP brands specifically labeled for birth control (Orgametril, Lutényl) are not yet available in the United States. But there are other mini pills available here, as well as full-dose brands that can be used for period control (so we'll restrict our discussion of full-dose POPs to those used for menstrual management). (Consult with your physician if you're interested in using full-dose POPs for birth control.)

For the most part, the same progestins that are used in combination birth control pills are also used in POPs. What's different is the amount of progestin: mini-dose POPs usually have less progestins, while full-dose POPs have more, compared to combination pills. Because of the different dosages and types of progestin used, the full-dose POPs have somewhat of a different profile—who can and can't use them, advantages and disadvantages—compared to the mini-dose POPs. What follows is a discussion of the mini-pill characteristics. For more detailed information on the full-dose POPs, consult your physician or visit www.tcoyp.com.

Who Can Use Progestin-Only Pills (POPs)?

You can use POPs if you:

* *Can't or don't want to use estrogen.* If you cannot tolerate estrogen or you have a health condition—such as abnormally thick uterine lining (endometrial hyperplasia) or breast problems—that would be made worse by estrogen, then POPs are a good option.

* *Are breastfeeding.* Not only are POPs safe during breastfeeding but they actually appear to promote breast milk production.

* *Smoke and are 35 years or older.*

* *Are perimenopausal.* "Perimenopause" refers to the transition years leading to menopause. The length of perimenopause differs from woman to woman—from one to nine years, but is usually around four years. During this time many women experience a variety of problems, like irregular periods, skin breakouts, and hot flashes. Conditions like endometriosis and fibroids tend to flare up.

* *Have a history of blood clot problems (thromboembolic disease).*

* *Have risk factors for breast cancer.*

* *Have a seizure disorder.*

* *Have a connective tissue disease, like lupus.*

* *Have certain liver conditions.* You may still be able to use POPs if you have chronic liver disease or if you developed jaundice while being pregnant or while taking combination pills.

* *Have high blood pressure (hypertension) or migraine headaches.*

* *Have blood sugar problems (altered glucose tolerance, including diabetes mellitus).*

Who Cannot Use Progestin-Only Pills (POPs)?

For legal rather than scientific reasons, POP brands in the United States carry the same contraindications as combination pills. However, POPs have a different user profile than combination pill brands.

Do not use POPs if you have any of the following conditions:

* **Known or suspected pregnancy.**

* **An allergy to any of the Pill's components.**

* **A history of, or very high risk for, arterial blood vessel disease.**

* **Active, severe liver disease.**

* **Known or suspected uterine or breast cancer.**

* **Abnormal genital bleeding (e.g., from the uterus or vagina).** Don't start using the Pill until the cause of the abnormal bleeding has been diagnosed and treated.

You should use POPs with caution if you have any of the following conditions:

* **A personal history of breast cancer.**

* **A history of ectopic pregnancy.**

* **A history of noncancerous ovarian cysts.**

* **A history of serious side effects not clearly attributable to estrogen while using combination pills.** Some women who use the combination pill can develop a problem like liver adenoma (a noncancerous growth) or cholestasis (a blockage in the flow of bile that can lead to jaundice). Because it's not clear that the estrogen in the combination pill is the culprit, it's better not to use a pill method at all.

* **A history of high blood pressure (hypertension) or migraines while using combination pills.**

* **Recent trophoblastic disease.** Trophoblastic disease is a condition seen in pregnant women or women who have been pregnant. Very briefly, what happens is that there's an abnormal growth (inside the uterus and throughout the body) of the tissues formed as a result of conception. Women who have this disease must not become pregnant for at least one year after they are treated. Because POPs are not as effective at preventing pregnancy as other methods, it's better to avoid using them during this time. The preferred birth control methods are combination pills or the injectable Depo-Provera.

* **A history of gestational diabetes, and you're a breastfeeding Latina.** One study found that Latina women who developed diabetes during their pregnancies (gestational diabetes), and who were breastfeeding and used POPs, had a significantly increased risk of developing permanent type 2 diabetes.

* **You're using liver enzyme–inducing drugs.** If you take certain drugs, like barbiturates, antibiotics (rifampin), or antiseizure medications (carbamazepine, phenytoin), it's best not to use POPs (or implants, for that matter). That's because these drugs lower the blood levels of the hormone in POPs. This may reduce the pregnancy protection, and it could also increase the likelihood of irregular bleeding. The preferred methods for you are Depo-Provera (an injection) and the hormone-releasing intrauterine device (IUD).

Advantages of Using Progestin-Only Pills (POPs)

You can use POPs to manage your menstrual period. Although POPs are not a first-choice method when it comes to menstrual management (for reasons we'll discuss shortly), they do, nonetheless, offer benefits. Women who use POPs have lighter bleeding episodes or even none at all. In particular, this method can help women with:

* *Painful and/or heavy, prolonged periods (dysmenorrhea and/or menorrhagia)*

* Premenstrual symptoms (PMS)

* Pain at the time of ovulation (mittelschmerz)

* Endometriosis

* Menstrual migraines

* Anemia

Just like the combination pill, POPs offer you a number of health benefits unrelated to their ability to prevent a pregnancy. For example, POPs:

* Offer some protection against ovarian and uterine cancers.

* Provide some protection against pelvic inflammatory disease (PID). Because POPs work by thickening the cervical mucus, there's less chance for bacteria to go up from the vagina into the uterus. However, if you're sexually active, you shouldn't rely on POPs to protect you from sexually transmitted infections (STIs). Certain barrier methods, like the condom, offer the best protection.

* Are less likely to increase blood pressure or cause headaches.

* Do not increase the risk of heart or blood vessel disease.

* Have minimal effect on metabolism. You can use mini-dose POPs even if you have liver problems, problems with cholesterol or sugar metabolism, or problems with blood sugar.

* Tend to cause less skin discoloration (chloasma) than the combination pill.

* May improve depression.

Disadvantages of Using Progestin-Only Pills (POPs)

Because POPs do not have estrogen, the side effects are different from the side effects of combination pills. Since the hormone comes in the form of a pill, POPs also tend to have slightly different disadvantages from other progestin-only methods that are administered by a different route, like shots or implants.

The main disadvantages of POPs are:

* *Irregular bleeding (most common)*. It's common for women who use POPs to experience bleeding irregularities. For example, it's estimated that 30 percent of women who use the full-dose pill experience this problem. Some of these bleeding irregularities are breakthrough bleeding or spotting, increased bleeding, and no bleeding at all (amenorrhea). Of course, if you use POPs for menstrual management, the lack of bleeding is a feature, not a flaw. However, for many women irregular bleeding makes the POP a less attractive method of menstrual management.

* *Increased incidence of noncancerous (functional) ovarian cysts.*

* *Very tight dosing window (older brands)*. This applies particularly to the older mini-pill brands. In order for those brands to provide maximal pregnancy protection, as well as reduce the likelihood of irregular bleeding, the pill had to be taken at the same time each day. If you took a pill even three hours later than the schedule time, you had to use a backup method of birth control, and you were more likely to experience irregular bleeding.

* *Less effective pregnancy protection than the combination pill (not all brands)*. This problem is especially true with the older mini-dose brands that do not consistently inhibit the release of the egg from the ovary (ovulation).

* *Increased likelihood of ectopic pregnancy*. If you take POPs your overall risk of an ectopic pregnancy is decreased (compared to women who don't use any birth control). However, if you do become pregnant while using POPs, the pregnancy is more likely to be ectopic. That's because the hormone in POPs alters the fallopian tube movement, which can cause the egg to become stuck in the tube.

For a list of progesterone-related side effects, see page 146.

How Do You Use Progestin-Only Pills (POPs)?

Before we see how the POP is used to manage your period, remember that there are two types of POPs: the mini-dose pill and the full-dose pill. Both types can be used for birth control or for menstrual management and both types are monophasic—all the pills in a given pack contain hormones (all are active) and all have the same amount of hormone. Most mini-pill brands come in 28-day packs; most of the full-dose brands come in 20-day packs.

THE BIRTH CONTROL REGIMEN

Although both the mini-dose and the full-dose POPs can be used for birth control, we'll restrict our discussion here to the mini-pill brands. (If you're interested in using a full-dose brand for birth control, consult with your physician or visit www.tcoyp.com.)

Most mini-pill brands come in 28-day packs. When you use this pill for birth control you take a pill once a day, at the same time each day, until the pack is used up. During the last seven days of the pack, most women have a bleeding episode.

When you first start using the POP, you'll usually begin on the first day of the menstrual cycle ("Day 1" start). It usually takes between seven and fourteen days (depending on which brand you use) for this method to offer full birth control protection. So, if you're sexually active, when you first start taking the POP, you need to use a backup method (like a barrier method) for seven to fourteen days.

POPs have a very tight dosing schedule—you have to take the pill at the same time each day. If you deviate from the timetable even by as little as three hours (for the older brands) the pregnancy protection diminishes. Your likelihood of experiencing irregular bleeding or spotting is also increased. To limit the irregular bleeding, if you forget to take a pill, take the missed pill as soon as you remember, and then take the next pill at the regularly scheduled time. Continue to take the remaining pills in the pill pack to avoid irregular bleeding for that month. (If you're sexually active, you need to use a backup birth control method. Consult with your physician for the details.)

Bottom line: when you use POPs for birth control you typically have lighter and less bleeding and, for some women, no bleeding at all.

THE MENSTRUAL MANAGEMENT REGIMEN

Based on your menstrual management end goals, the POP regimens used fall into two broad groups: passive and active.

Passive period control regimen:

This regimen works best if one of these is your end goal:

* Reducing the amount and duration of bleeding

* Reducing the number of bleeding episodes, or possibly stopping the monthly bleeding altogether

For example, this regimen will help:

* If you have heavy, week-long periods and you'd like to have lighter, shorter bleeding

* If you suffer from period-related problems

The regular birth control regimen can help you achieve any of these goals. You take the POP the same way as if you were using it for pregnancy protection—one pill, at the same time each day, for twenty-eight days in a row. Of course, just because you're using birth control, that doesn't mean you have to actually be sexually active.

For this type of regimen, you can use any mini-pill POP brand. However, usually the best choices are the newer mini-pill brands, like Cerazette, and the full-dose ones. (If you're using a full-dose brand for birth control, check with your physician for the regimen.) The reason you can use this regimen is because of the way the POP works. Overall, women who use POPs have lighter monthly bleeding than do women who use the combination pill for birth control (the regular, 21/7 regimen). Moreover, some women who use POPs no longer have a monthly period. For example, 20 percent of women who use a particular brand of mini pill stop having periods. Of course, since this is passive management, you can't actually control whether you're one of the 20 percent.

The main advantage of using this POP regimen is that women who don't want to take or can't tolerate estrogen can use it. For example, if you're breastfeeding, if you suffer from breast problems or a thickened uterine lining (endometrial hyperplasia), or if you are a smoker over the age of 35, you can safely use POPs. In addition, POPs (especially the full-dose brands) can help perimenopausal women and women with premenstrual symptoms (PMS), hot flashes, heavy periods (due to uterine fibroids or a thickened endometrium), painful periods (dysmenorrhea), breast pain (mastalgia), and noncancerous breast tumors (fibroadenomas).

Of course, if you can use POPs you can also use other types of progestin-only methods, like shots, implants, and intrauterine devices (IUDs) as an alternative menstrual management method. (We'll discuss these methods shortly.)

As we mentioned at the start of this section, the passive regimen is not the first choice when it comes to menstrual management. That's because the main side effect of using POPs is bleeding irregularities—spotting, early or late bleeding, and even an increased flow. In other words, not only can't you control whether you bleed, but you also can't regulate the bleeding. Although you'll bleed less frequently or maybe not at all, the bleeding will still most likely be irregular. The problem is it's not possible to predict which women will experience which pattern. This is also why, if you're interested in using this method, it's best to give it a trial run—at least six months—before deciding how often and for how long to use it. Once you have an idea of what your particular bleeding pattern is while using POPs, you'll be in a better position to evaluate whether the method is right for you. In general, even for women interested in passive period management, other progestin-only methods might be better options because they produce fewer bleeding irregularities.

Active period control regimen:

Think of the POP active period control management as less of a regimen and more of a "quick intervention force," used to quickly stop or postpone the period. For example, this regimen is used if you have a particularly heavy, prolonged period and are anemic and need to stop the loss of blood as soon as possible. It can also be used to postpone a period, or shift the cycle schedule, so you can avoid having a period during a particular time.

This is a high-dose regimen using full-dose pills. The schedule and number of pills you take depends on which brand you use. Usually, to postpone the period, a continuous regimen is used: one pill is taken one to three times a day, starting two weeks (or even one week) before the scheduled start of the period. A different regimen—this one cyclical—involves starting to take a pill on the fifth day of the menstrual cycle.

For this cyclical regimen, usually one pill is taken for twenty days, preferably at the same time each day. Then no pills are taken for ten days, after which a new pack is started. Most women experience an episode of bleeding during the pill-free days. Some of the progestins used are: lynestrenol (Orgametril) and norethisterone (norethindrone) acetate (Primolut Nor). Remember, these are full-dose brands, and the active POP regimen involves much higher doses than those in the passive, mini-pill POP regimen.

As a result, you're more likely to experience side effects like breast tenderness or nausea, which limits the long-term use of these full-dose regimens. For example, a study that found that a high-dose POP regimen reduced period blood loss by 87 percent also found that only 22 percent of women expressed interest in continuing to use the regimen. The active POP method is best reserved for medical problems and occasional lifestyle use—if you need to postpone your period on short notice for an important event, as opposed to every other month. Your physician will be able to go over the details.

The bottom line: if you want to use menstrual management for lifestyle issues (you lead an active lifestyle), POPs are not a good option for you. However, for women who need period control to benefit their health and who can't or don't want to use any of the other available hormonal methods, POPs offer a valuable alternative.

Cerazette

Cerazette is a newer mini-dose progestin-only pill (POP) brand that is not yet available in the United States. It contains 0.075 milligrams of the progestin desogestrel and it comes in a 28-day pack. All the pills in the pack are active (all have hormones) and you take one pill per day, preferably at the same time each day.

The advantage of using this pill is that about 20 percent of the women who use it as birth control stop bleeding altogether or have infrequent episodes of spotting. This is listed as a side effect in the package insert, but, of course, it becomes an advantage for women who don't want to bleed every month, or for whom the bleeding is problematic for their health.

The particular disadvantage of using this pill brand is that there's no way to predict in advance which women will stop bleeding while using it.

Resource: http://www.organon.com/products/contraception/cerazette.asp (site maintained by the manufacturer).

See Appendix A for a sample list of mini-dose and full-dose brands of progestin-only pills.

Let's turn our attention now to the three remaining passive menstrual management methods:

* Shots

* Implants

* Hormone-releasing intrauterine devices (IUDs)

All these methods contain hormones—some have both an estrogen and a progestin, while others have only a progestin. They are all long-acting methods. Depending on which method you choose, you can use it continuously for anywhere from one month to five years. The hormones are slowly released into the body and work over months or years. Overall, if you use implants, shots, or hormonal IUDs you can expect to have less frequent bleeding, decreased flow, or even no bleeding at all. The drawback is that you have little, if any, control over the timing and pattern of bleeding. Two features make these methods unsuitable for active management: the way they're administered and their ability to work for a long time. For example, it's just not practical to have an implant inserted and removed (minor office procedures) every few months. Also, once a shot has been administered it takes the body some time to clear the hormones (not just twenty-four hours as with the Pill).

The good news is that many women can benefit from menstrual management by using shots, implants, and/or hormonal IUDs. In particular, if you can't or don't want to use any of the other methods, any of these three long-term hormonal methods is an option. And, of course, for sexually active women who prefer to have little involvement with their birth control method, something like an IUD—in and "out of mind" for five years—might even be preferable to the other period control methods.

Let's now look at the three long-acting methods in more detail, particularly at their use in menstrual management.

Shots

There are two types of hormonal birth control shots (injections), just as there are two types of birth control pills:

* One-hormone shots (progestin-only shots)

* Two-hormone shots (combination estrogen and progestin)

Most of our discussion will concentrate on the progestin-only group for two reasons: it can be used for menstrual management, and it's the only one available to women in the United States.

Progestin-Only Shot

As the name implies, this shot contains only one hormone—a progestin. The type and dose of progestin vary, depending on which brand you use. The shot is administered by medical personnel every two to three months and has been available worldwide since the 1970s. In 1992 it became available in the United States.

Because the hormone is injected, the women who can and can't use it and its advantages and disadvantages differ slightly from the ones for the progestin-only pill.

Who Can Use the Progestin-Only Shot?

You can use the progestin-only shot if you:

* *Are a good candidate for hormonal birth control pills.* And you:

- Cannot, or do not want to, remember to take a pill every day.
- Want to use a hormonal method but experienced minor side effects while taking the combination pill or the progestin-only pill.

Also, you can use this method if you:

* *Do not want to use or can't tolerate estrogen.* You can use this method if you cannot use estrogen because you have risk factors for any of the following:

- Blood clots
- Stroke
- Coronary artery disease (the blood vessels that supply the heart)
- Migraines
- Diabetes
- Systemic lupus erythematosus (an autoimmune disease)

* *Suffer from any of these medical conditions:*

• Venous thromboembolism or varicose veins (While the package insert lists thromboembolic disease [blood clots and their complications] as a contraindication, there's little scientific evidence to back this claim.)
• Epilepsy
• Hyperlipidemia (an excess of fats in the blood)
• Mild diabetes (Depo-Provera has a slight tendency to increase blood sugar so use with caution if you're a diabetic.)
• Sickle-cell disease
• Tuberculosis
• Malaria and/or schistosomiasis (a tropical disease caused by a parasite)

The progestin-only shot can also be used by women who:

* *Have just given birth.*

* *Are breastfeeding (especially the first six weeks after delivery).* There is extensive clinical experience with the use of progestin-only shots in breastfeeding women. This birth control method does not affect milk production or infant weight gain.

* *Smoke and are over the age of 35.*

* *Want a very effective method that requires minimal user involvement.*

* *Want to delay pregnancy for several years but want to have children at a later date.*

Who Cannot Use the Progestin-Only Shot?

Do not use the progestin-only shot if you have any of the following conditions:

* **Known or suspected pregnancy.**

* **An allergy to any of the shot's components.**

* Current breast cancer.

* Abnormal genital bleeding (e.g., from the uterus or vagina).

* Active liver diseases or liver tumors.

* You're planning a pregnancy within two years.

If you have any of the following conditions, it's best to use another method, like the progestin-only pill:

* Stroke, or severe recurrent headaches associated with difficulty seeing, speaking, or moving.

* Severe high blood pressure (hypertension).

* Ischemic heart disease (disease caused by blocked arteries).

* Severe diabetes.

* A history of breast cancer.

* If you're sexually active and take medicine (aminoglutethimide) for Cushing's disease (a hormonal condition).

Advantages of Using the Progestin-Only Shot

You can use the progestin-only shot to manage your menstrual period. Women who use the progestin-only shot are less likely to have heavy monthly bleeding, and quite a number of users stop having periods altogether. For example, 50 percent of women who use Depo-Provera no longer have periods after the first year of use. This number goes up to 75 percent over the long run. Some of the problems this method can help with are:

* *Painful periods*

* *Premenstrual symptoms, like PMS*

* *Endometriosis*

* *Seizures*

Progestin-only shots offer a number of nonpregnancy-related benefits, such as:

* *Markedly reduced risk of uterine cancer (up to 80 percent).*

* *Reduced frequency of crises in women with sickle-cell disease.*

* *Reduced seizure episodes in women with epilepsy.*

* *No increase in the risk of ovarian, cervical, or breast cancer.*

* *Reduced incidence of pelvic inflammatory disease (PID) and yeast infections.* (Depo-Provera offers some protection against PID because the cervical mucus is thickened and thus the bacteria may have a harder time passing through into the cervix. However, if you're sexually active, you shouldn't rely on this method to protect you from sexually transmitted infections [STIs]. Use a barrier method for STI protection.)

Disadvantages of Using the Progestin-Only Shot

Irregular bleeding (main side effect):
When you use this method, especially Depo-Provera, bleeding disturbances—spotting and breakthrough bleeding, absence of bleeding (amenorrhea), and, less commonly, heavy bleeding—are the rule rather than the exception. These side effects may persist months after this method is stopped. Because of the way the hormone is released, it takes about six to eight months after the last shot for its effects on your bleeding pattern to subside.

Potential negative impact on bone density:
Some studies have shown no significant effect of the progestin-only shot on bone health. In other studies, Depo-Provera was found to decrease bone mass to some degree. (The greatest loss happens when you first start using it, especially if you're an adolescent or a young woman. This loss slows over time.) The bone loss appears to be almost completely reversible once you stop using the method, even after long-term use (four years or more). The degree and re-

versibility of bone loss with Depo-Provera are comparable to those seen in breastfeeding women. This suggests that a long-term increase in osteoporosis (brittle bones) risk in Depo-Provera users is unlikely.

Decreased "good" cholesterol (HDL) levels:
"Bad" cholesterol (LDL) has been linked to narrowing of the blood vessels (atherosclerosis), while "good" cholesterol (HDL) reduces the risk of atherosclerosis. Atherosclerosis is a major cause of heart attack, stroke, and other vascular disease. The progestin-only shot reduces HDL in long-term users, but LDL is not increased. You should not use this method if you have severe vascular disease (such as severe hypertension, a history of stroke, or ischemic heart disease) or diabetes involving vascular complications. If you develop these conditions while using the progestin-only shot or if you develop recurrent severe headaches associated with difficulty seeing, speaking, or moving, you should see a physician immediately and switch to a nonhormonal method.

Slight tendency to increase blood sugar:
Progestin-only injectables don't induce diabetes in healthy women, but they slightly increase blood sugar and insulin levels in long-term users.

Lag time between stopping the method and return of fertility:
Once you stop using this method, the average time for fertility to return is ten months, but it can be as long as twenty-two months. After the final shot, 68 percent of women will be able to conceive during the first year, 83 percent within fifteen months, and 93 percent within eighteen months. Obviously, if you want to use menstrual management but plan to become pregnant in the near future, it's best to use another method.

Increased relative risk of ectopic pregnancy:
If you use the progestin-only shot, your risk of an ectopic pregnancy is decreased (compared to women who don't use birth con-

trol). However, if you do become pregnant while using this method, there's a higher chance that the pregnancy will be ectopic.

Weight:

The popular wisdom is that Depo-Provera leads to significant weight gain, especially over time. However, studies have disproved this; no specific relationship between Depo-Provera and change in weight or in the balance of food intake to energy expenditure has been documented.

Does this mean that it's a sure thing that you'll stay svelte while using the progestin-only shot? Unfortunately, no. Some women gain weight; others don't. For example, an uncontrolled study of Depo-Provera users noted that 60 percent of women gained weight during the first six months of use. The degree of weight gain was five pounds after one year, and fifteen pounds after three years. However, women who don't use any birth control also tend to gain weight over time. The bottom line is that even though the product insert lists weight gain as a possible side effect, there isn't conclusive scientific evidence supporting this link. If you do experience weight gain while using Depo-Provera you can always switch to another method.

Mood changes:

Some women who use Depo-Provera may experience mood changes, like depression, while others don't. However, studies have not shown that this method increases depressive symptoms, even in women who complained of this problem before starting to use the method.

For a list of progesterone-related side effects see page 146.

How Do You Use Progestin-Only Shots?

The progestin-only shot is administered in a doctor's office. One shot lasts for two to three months, depending on which brand you use. The shot is administered as an intramuscular injection in the arm, thigh, or buttock. During the months between shots, the hormone slowly diffuses out of the muscle and into the bloodstream. This is called the depot intramuscular route.

Usually, the same regimen used for birth control is also used for menstrual management.

Let's take a closer look at the two brands of progestin-only shots—Depo-Provera and Noristerat—their regimens, and what they can do for you when it comes to menstrual management.

Depo-Provera

Depo-Provera is a shot that contains 150 milligrams of the progestin medroxyprogesterone acetate. The hormone comes in "depot" form—it's released slowly, over months. (Hence, the medical name for this shot: depot medroxyprogesterone acetate, or DMPA.) Other brand names for this shot are Depo-Ralovera and Depo-Clinovir.

THE BIRTH CONTROL REGIMEN

The Depo-Provera birth control regimen is one 150-milligram shot, given once every three months (only four times a year). Ideally, the first shot is given within the first five days after the start of your menstrual period. It's best if the next injection is not delayed by more than one week—the birth control protection could be decreased, but, more important for our discussion, the likelihood of irregular bleeding or spotting will be increased.

THE MENSTRUAL MANAGEMENT REGIMEN

Depo-Provera will work best for you if your period control goals are to:

* Significantly reduce the amount, frequency, and duration of bleeding

* Stop having periods altogether

Half of the women who use Depo-Provera stop having periods during the first year of use; over the long run the number increases to 75 percent.

For example, this regimen will help if:

* Your menstrual period is heavy, or it lasts long enough to cause serious medical problems.

* You'd like to, or need to, stop having periods altogether.

Usually, the same regimen used for birth control—one 150-milligram shot, once every three months—is also used for menstrual management. To obtain the best results in terms of period suppression it's best to have the shot within the first five days after the start of the period, and no later than Day 10 to 13 of the menstrual cycle. Some other regimens used are giving the next shot early—usually every eight to ten weeks (although a study didn't find this regimen more effective)—or giving a 300-milligram shot once every one to three months. The higher-dose regimens have somewhat different side effects. They can't be used long-term because of possible increased negative effect on bone density. Your physician will be able to go over the advantages and disadvantages of the various regimens.

There are two main advantages of using Depo-Provera for menstrual management. First, women who don't want to or can't use other methods, especially the estrogen-containing ones, can use this method. In particular, women who suffer from seizure disorders and/or medical diseases like lupus or who are HIV-positive can safely use Depo-Provera. Second, a large number of women who use this method long-term stop having periods altogether.

The disadvantage of using Depo-Provera for menstrual management is that you can't control your bleeding pattern. For example, although you'll most likely stop having periods after the first few shots, it's not possible to predict in advance if and when this will happen. (Usually, the lack of periods is uncommon in the first few months of use and it becomes progressively more likely with time.)

Another disadvantage is the fact that the effects of the shot on the bleeding pattern tend to continue for at least six to eight months after you're given the last shot. You basically have no way of controlling when the bleeding starts or stops with this method.

If you want to use menstrual management for lifestyle issues (you lead an active lifestyle, you have an upcoming special event) or for short-term purposes, Depo-Provera is not a good option for you. However, for women whose period can cause health problems and/or for those who suffer from a number of medical diseases, Depo-Provera is a very good passive menstrual management option.

Resource: http://www.Depo-Provera.com (site maintained by the manufacturer).

Noristerat

Noristerat (Norigest, Noristat) is the other progestin-only birth control shot. It contains 200 milligrams of the progestin norethindrone (norethisterone) enanthate (NET-EN). Another brand name for this shot is Doryxas; Noristerat isn't available yet in the United States.

THE BIRTH CONTROL REGIMEN

When Noristerat is used for birth control, one shot is given every two months. An alternative regimen is one shot every two months for six months and then one shot every three months. It's best to have the first injection within the first seven days after the start of the period. Also, it's best not to delay the next injection for more than one week to decrease the likelihood of irregular bleeding or spotting.

THE MENSTRUAL MANAGEMENT REGIMEN

Noristerat will work best for you if your period goals are to:

* Significantly reduce the amount, frequency, and duration of bleeding

* Regulate your periods

For example, this regimen will help if:

* Your menstrual period is heavy or lasts long enough to cause serious medical problems.

* You'd like your bleeding to be more regular.

The same regimen used for birth control—one 200-milligram shot, once every two months—is also used for menstrual management. To obtain the best results in terms of period inhibition it's best to have the shot within the first seven days after the start of the period.

Although, overall, Noristerat is similar to Depo-Provera, and most women experience similar bleeding irregularities with both, there are two differences that might make it a better option for some women.

First, the bleeding irregularities experienced by women using Noristerat are of a lower intensity. In particular, if you use this method you're less likely to experience prolonged bleeding or spotting during the first six months. Second, fewer women stop having periods completely after one year—about a third of women using Noristerat, compared with about half of Depo-Provera users. So, if you're a woman interested in menstrual management who prefers to have some monthly bleeding, Noristerat may be a better choice for you.

The particular disadvantages of using this method are that it's an oil-based shot, which makes it a more painful injection, and the fact that you need to have a shot more often, which could make it more expensive.

Resource: http://www.fhi.org/training/en/modules/INJ/s3pg1.htm (site maintained by Family Health International).

Two-Hormone Shot

The other group of hormonal injections is the combination shot, which has two hormones—an estrogen and a progestin. The shot is administered by medical personnel, and many brands have been available worldwide for years except in the United States. In 2000, one brand, Lunelle, medroxyprogesterone acetate and estradiol cypionate (MPA/E2C) briefly became available in the United States. In October 2002, Lunelle was voluntarily recalled from the U.S. market (because of plant manufacturing problems) and, as of the time of this writing, there are no plans to reintroduce it. Regrettably, since Lunelle was the only combination shot available in the United States, once again American women are left without an alternative.

Because the combination shot has an estrogen and a progestin just as the other combination methods (the Pill, the skin patch, and the vaginal ring) do, its general profile—who can and can't use it (see pages 139–141), and advantages and disadvantages (see pages 141–152)—are similar. Obviously, there are also some specific advantages (you don't have to remember to take a pill every day) and disadvantages (discomfort at injection site).

How Do You Use the Combination Shot?

Just like the progestin-only shot, the combination shot is administered in a doctor's office. For most brands, one shot lasts for one month. The shot is administered as an intramuscular injection in the arm or the buttock. During the month, the hormone slowly diffuses out of the muscle and into the bloodstream.

THE BIRTH CONTROL REGIMEN
This shot is administered in the arm or buttocks, usually as a monthly injection. The type and dose of hormones vary, depending on the brand used. Check with your physician for the exact regimen.

THE MENSTRUAL MANAGEMENT REGIMEN
The combination shot is a good option if your menstrual management goals are to:

* Reduce the amount, frequency, and duration of bleeding

* Regulate your periods

For example, the combination shot can help if:

* Your menstrual period is heavy and lasts long enough to cause serious medical problems.

* Your cycles are irregular and you'd like to bleed at predictable intervals.

Usually, the same regimen used for birth control is used for menstrual management—one shot monthly. So far, for Lunelle, there's no evidence indicating that changing the injection interval (having the shot at more frequent intervals than four weeks) will result in no more monthly bleeding (amenorrhea).

The main advantage of using the combination shot is that two-thirds of users experience a predictable monthly fake period. In addition, women who use this method have a lower number of bleeding days per cycle, relative to a natural cycle.

The drawback of the combination shot is that one of the main side effects of this method is bleeding irregularities: spotting, bleeding more days than usual, no periods at all. For example, during the first three to six months of use, about 24 percent of women experience some form of irregular bleeding and 4 percent develop prolonged bleeding. Of course, another disadvantage of this method is that you don't have control over the bleeding pattern—once you have the shot, you can't predict beforehand what will happen.

If you can use estrogen, the other estrogen methods (the Pill, skin patch, and vaginal ring) are preferable to the combination shot because they allow you to actively manage your period. However, if you can accept the limitations of a passive method, and you don't mind having a monthly fake period, the combination shot might be a good option for you.

Resources: http://www.Lunelle.com (site maintained by manufacturer).

Implants

The implant is a hormonal method of birth control that comes in the form of one or several small plastic rods, or a capsule. Each rod has a small amount of only one hormone, a progestin. The number of rods, and the amount and type of progestin, depend on which brand of implant you use. The rods are inserted and removed by medical personnel. Used since 1983, implants are widely available world-wide, except in the United States. They were approved and became available for use in the United States in 1990, but in 2002 the distribution of the only available brand, Norplant, was stopped. American women are once again deprived of an entire group of methods.

Who Can Use Implants?

Anyone who can use progestin-only pills can use implants. (See page 180.)

Who Cannot Use Implants?

Anyone who can't use progestin-only pills should not use implants. (See pages 181–182 for disqualifying and cautionary factors.)

Advantages of Using Implants

The advantages of using implants are almost identical to those for the progestin-only pill. Some of the unique advantages of implants include:

* *Lower likelihood of causing bleeding irregularities.* If you use implants you have less bleeding compared to real menstrual periods. It's possible to experience bleeding irregularities; however, by the end of one year most implant users (who use the newer brands) tend to have a regular, monthly bleeding pattern.

* *No effect on bone density.* Unlike the progestin-only shot, implants have no effect on bones; they don't cause bone loss.

* *Highly effective, long-term, reversible protection against pregnancy.* The implant is one of the most effective methods of birth control—better than sterilization! The first-year failure rates are 0 percent (Implanon) to 0.05 percent (Norplant and Jadelle) for both perfect and typical use, whereas the failure rate for sterilization is 0.4 percent.

Implants also don't require any maintenance, and they don't interfere with the spontaneity of sexual intercourse. In addition, the daily hormone dose is lower than in other methods and fertility returns as soon as you stop using the method. Once the implant is removed, its hormones are cleared in five days (Norplant) to one week (Implanon).

Disadvantages of Using Implants

The disadvantages of using implants are almost identical to those for the progestin-only pill. The notable differences are:

Headaches (common side effect):
Approximately 10–30 percent of women who use this method complain of headaches. However, less than 5 percent of women discontinue using the implant because of headache.

Insertion and removal require a physician, and a minor surgical procedure is performed at the doctor's office.

Insertion site complications:
In a small number of women, bruising, swelling, discomfort, and, rarely, infection may develop at the insertion site. Even less common is expulsion of the implant. For example, the incidence of infection or expulsion following insertion varies from none to 0.5 percent of insertions.

Problems with removal (older brands):

For the older brands (Norplant), removal can be uncomfortable and more difficult than insertion if scar tissue has formed over the implants. Removal usually takes 15 to 20 minutes but it may take longer and require more than one visit. The reported percentages of removal complications have ranged between 0.2 percent and 7.0 percent. This is not a problem with the newer brands because they have fewer rods than the older ones. Studies that compare Norplant with the newer brands, Implanon and Jadelle, have shown significantly reduced rates of removal complications with the two newer systems. The removal procedure takes less time for Implanon and Jadelle than for Norplant—5.4 minutes for Implanon versus Norplant's 15 to 20 minutes.

Decreased effectiveness with some medications:

If you're sexually active and you're taking certain medications—barbiturates, carbamazepine, phenytoin, and rifampin—the implant's pregnancy protection effectiveness is reduced.

Weight:

As with Depo-Provera, women using implants (4–22 percent of all users) report weight gain of 0.9 to 3.3 pounds (0.4–1.5 kg) per year. However, just because some women gain weight while using this method, that doesn't automatically mean the implant is the culprit. For example, one study reported similar weight gains between implant users and women who weren't using a hormonal method, while another study showed a small (0.4 pounds, or 0.2 kg, per year) increase in weight in Norplant users.

✻ DEFINITION

The failure rate is the number of pregnancies per 100 woman-years. In other words, if a method has a 5 percent failure rate, out of 100 woman who used that method, five would be pregnant within one year. Perfect use means the method is used exactly as it's supposed to be used; typical use means real life use, where mistakes sometimes happen.

Mood changes:

Between 1 percent and 9 percent of women using implants report mood changes, like depression or nervousness. However, studies don't show a direct cause-and-effect association.

How Do You Use Implants?

THE BIRTH CONTROL REGIMEN

The implant is inserted under the skin, usually in the underarm of the nondominant arm. This is done during an office visit and the procedure takes just a few minutes. Depending on the brand, an implant lasts from six months to five years. The hormone in the implant slowly diffuses out into the body, a little bit at a time, over years (for most brands). At the end of the use interval (or sooner, if you wish) the implant is removed (also during an office visit). Like insertion, removal takes only a few minutes.

THE MENSTRUAL MANAGEMENT REGIMEN

Implants, in particular the newer brands, can benefit you if your main menstrual management goals are to:

* Reduce the frequency of bleeding and, to a lesser extent, the amount

* Regulate the bleeding

For example, this method is helpful if:

* You have prolonged and heavy periods and you want to bleed less, and less often.

* You're interested in both period control and long-term birth control.

The same regimen used for birth control is also used for menstrual management. For more details, see the sections about the individual methods.

There are several advantages to using implants for menstrual management. Women who don't want to use or can't tolerate estrogen can use implants. Also, women who either want or need to have less frequent bleeding, or none at all, can use this method. For example, a significant number of women who use Implanon experience infrequent bleeding and/or none at all. One study found that, by the end of the first year of use, up to three-quarters of the women had a normal regular bleeding pattern. Finally, implants are also very convenient if you're interested in long-term menstrual management, especially if you're sexually active.

There is one main drawback to using implants for period control: you have to be patient. Bleeding disturbances—irregular and prolonged (but not heavier) bleeding—are almost the rule, especially in the first few months of use. With Norplant or Jadelle, prolonged or irregular bleeding is common during the first year of use; with Implanon, irregular bleeding is common in the first months of use. Although for all brands, bleeding patterns improve with time, you have to be willing to wait.

Another obvious disadvantage of implants is the fact that, once the implant is in, you have no way of regulating the bleeding pattern. It's impractical, not to mention possibly expensive, to have the implant inserted and removed too frequently.

If you're interested in short-term, lifestyle-oriented menstrual management, implants are not the best option for you. If you must use a progestin-only method, the progestin-only pill or the hormone-releasing IUD might be a better option. However, implants are very useful for women who want or need to decrease the frequency of bleeding as well as the amount of flow. Implants are also very good for women with any of the following health problems: endometriosis, anemia, or painful periods (dysmenorrhea).

About Specific Brands of Implants

There are several brands of implants available and, overall, their characteristics are similar. The main differences are between the older brands, like Norplant, and the relatively newer ones, like Implanon. So, let's briefly look at these two brands and highlight some of the differences, then take a quick look at some others.

NORPLANT

Norplant, the original six-rod implant, has been available since 1983 and is widely available worldwide, except in the United States. It has 216 milligrams of the progestin levonorgestrel and it releases about 85 micrograms per day in the first months of use, down to about 30 micrograms per day at the end of five years. This implant can be left in place for five years.

For women interested in menstrual management, the advantage of using this method is that about 6 percent of users will stop having periods altogether. However, this should be balanced with the fact that about 80 percent of users experience irregular bleeding, and the fact that this brand has six rods, which can make removal more difficult.

Resource: http://www.norplantinfo.com (site maintained by the manufacturer).

IMPLANON

Implanon is a newer implant brand that consists of one small rod that is about the size of a matchstick. It has 68 milligrams of the progestin etonogestrel and it releases an average of 40 micrograms per day. This implant can be used continuously for up to three years. Implanon is widely available in the United Kingdom and Europe, but it's not available in the United States yet.

There are several advantages to using Implanon. Up to 51 percent of women experience infrequent and/or regular bleeding after using it for one year. Also, you can use it to relieve period-related problems: over 85 percent of women with painful periods noted an improvement at the end of treatment, while 59 percent of women reported improved or disappearing acne. Finally, once you stop using this method and have the implant removed, the menstrual periods return to normal within three months.

The main disadvantage of using Implanon is irregular bleeding, which is most likely to happen during the first few months of use.

Resource: www.organon.com/products/contraception/implanon
.asp (site maintained by the manufacturer).

JADELLE (NORPLANT II)
This is an improved version of the original Norplant. Jadelle consists of only two rods, which are thinner and longer than the ones in the original Norplant. The rods have a total of 140 milligrams of the progestin levonorgestrel and may be used for up to five years. Jadelle is widely available worldwide but, although it is FDA-approved, it isn't yet available in the United States.
Resource: http://www.popcouncil.org/biomed/jadellefaq.html (site maintained by the Population Council).

NESTORONE
There are two types of implants that contain the progestin nestorone (old name ST1435). One implant consists of a single rod that releases 150 micrograms per day and lasts up to two years, while in another the hormone is contained in a small capsule that releases 45–50 micrograms per day and lasts for six months. The six-month system is available in Brazil under the brand name Elcometrine. It is used to treat endometriosis.

Hormone-Releasing Intrauterine Devices (IUDs)

The intrauterine device (IUD) is a small device that works inside the uterus. Worldwide, this is the most commonly used reversible method of birth control. IUDs require a doctor's prescription and many brands are available, except in the United States, where there are only two brands. IUDs have been known and used for thousands of years—three thousand years ago ancient traders used pebbles as an "IUD" for their camels so they wouldn't become pregnant during long trips, and the precursors of the modern devices have been around since the 1930s.

If there's a method that can be seen as the "poster child" of how misinformation prevents women from taking advantage of something that has tremendous potential to benefit them, it's the IUD. Much of the controversy has to do with the misperception surrounding the infection risk with IUD use and a lack of understanding of how the IUD works. The reality is that IUD users do not have a significantly higher risk of infection overall. Nor does the IUD work by destroying fertilized eggs. For those of you interested in a detailed discussion about IUDs' mechanism of action and the risk of infection associated with their use, see the box below. For everyone else, just know that an IUD may or may not be the best method for you, but you shouldn't allow misinformation to guide your health decisions.

There are many types of IUDs, but based on the overall design,

The IUD—Infection Risk and Mechanism of Action

The Dalkon Shield, a nonmedicated, framed IUD, was introduced in the United States in 1970. It had a plastic frame and an attached tail made of several filaments braided together (multifilament). In 1974 a report was published that described twelve cases of septic second-trimester abortions, five of which were fatal (the deaths were the result of infectious complications), in women using IUDs (a Dalkon Shield in ten cases, and a Lippes Loop in two). The report created suspicion that there might be something about the design of the Dalkon Shield that increased a woman's risk of widespread infection. After the report, the manufacturer of the Dalkon Shield suspended sales, and the sales were never resumed. Despite the fact that in October 1974 the FDA concluded that the safety of the Dalkon Shield was not significantly different from that of other IUD types, the manufacturer was sued and forced into bankruptcy.

During the lawsuits, a number of studies appeared that claimed a strong correlation between the use of an IUD and an increased risk of pelvic inflammatory disease (PID) in general—and an increased risk of PID in Dalkon Shield users in particular. Those studies were later discredited and their conclusions were shown to have been flawed.

So, what are the actual facts about IUD use and the risk of PID? A review of the largest IUD study database found that:

- **The overall rate of PID in IUD users was 1.6 cases per 1,000 women per year of use.**
- **The risk of PID was low and constant for up to eight years of follow-up.** In fact, long-term use of copper- and hormone-containing devices results in pelvic infection rates comparable to those of birth control pill users.
- **PID risk was more than six times higher during the twenty days after insertion than during later times.** (See discussion below.)

Another review article concluded that the risk of PID due to an intrauterine device is very low. In addition, even studies in which the rate of STIs was high among the general population found that the estimated risk of PID due to IUD use was very low—only 0.15 percent (less than 1 in 600).

And this is what happens to your pelvic inflammatory disease (PID) risk when you use an IUD:

Women at low risk of acquiring sexually transmitted infections (STIs) have little increase in the risk of PID. The single most important risk factor for PID is having sexual intercourse with multiple sexual partners, or with a partner who has multiple partners (because this increases the woman's exposure to STIs). If your risk of acquiring an STI is low, so is your risk of developing PID while using an IUD.

Women infected with, or at risk for acquiring, an STI have an increased risk of PID. Women who acquire gonococcal or chlamydial infection (two common STIs) might have an increased risk of developing PID while using the IUD.

PID risk is highest during the twenty days after insertion (PID is an infrequent event beyond the first twenty days after insertion).

The PID risk is highest during the twenty days after insertion because that's when bacteria may be introduced into the uterus by the insertion process. The vagina is not sterile; it's normally full of bacteria. (Don't worry; as long as they stay in the vagina, they're not harmful.) In contrast, the uterus is sterile relative to the vagina. And the IUD and its insertion device are 100 percent sterile. Of course, in order for the sterile IUD to get from its sterile package to the sterile uterus, it has to pass through the vagina. During the insertion process, some of the vaginal bacteria may be introduced into the uterus, causing a localized inflammatory reaction (a normal body response), which usually resolves naturally. However, if a vaginal (or pelvic) infection is already present, the IUD insertion may introduce harmful bacteria into the uterus (or may aggravate an already existing pelvic infection), causing or worsening PID.

Because of the increased risk with insertion, it's best if you leave the IUD in place up to its maximum lifespan, rather than have it routinely taken out and reinserted earlier. (Of course, if you decide you want to stop using it, you can have the IUD removed at any time.)

PID that develops after the first month of IUD use (unrelated to the insertion process) is caused by an STI, not the IUD.

Even after the Dalkon Shield was recalled and the incorrect studies were exposed, due to the litigious climate particular to the United States, IUD manufacturers ceased distribution of IUDs in this country. One IUD brand was later reintroduced, and currently there are only two types of IUDs available to American women—the ParaGard (TCu-380A) and Mirena. Less than 1 percent of American women use IUDs as a birth control method (sterilization is the most popular method). This is in contrast to the rest of the world, including third world nations, where the IUD is the most popular method of reversible birth control. The point is not that you should use the same birth control method used by women in other parts of the world. Rather, you should take a moment to ponder the reality that women in those countries, and pretty much everywhere else in the world, have far more birth control options than you do.

In light of all the misinformation and negative publicity about IUDs in the United States you'd think that no one in America likes this birth control method. Not true. The IUD is a favorite method used by women Ob/Gyns for their own birth control needs. Also the women who use it love it. Ninety-six percent of U.S. women using an IUD viewed their method of birth control favorably. By comparison, 94 percent of birth control pill users rated their method favorably, as did 93 percent of users of female and male sterilization, and 90 percent of condom users, while only 76 percent of diaphragm users and 74 percent of rhythm-method users had favorable views of their methods. But wait! That's not all the misinformation there is concerning the IUD. More often than not, the mechanism by which an IUD prevents pregnancy is misunderstood by women and health-care professionals alike.

The main mechanism by which IUDs offer pregnancy protection is by preventing the union of egg and sperm (fertilization). IUDs have a direct effect on sperm, killing them (IUDs are spermicidal). They also impede the movement of eggs, and the hormone-releasing IUDs thicken the cervical mucus, making it more difficult for sperm to get into the uterus. One additional mechanism, for the hormone-releasing brands, is the inhibition of ovulation. The progestin in these IUDs prevents the ovary from releasing an egg, by inhibiting the action of luteinizing hormone (LH).

The relationship between IUDs and pelvic inflammatory disease (PID) is often misunderstood and misstated, and so is the IUD's mechanism of action. This deprives you of options and keeps you from making an informed decision about something that has the potential to benefit your lifestyle and your health.

the two major groups are: framed and frameless IUDs. The frame devices have a small plastic frame, usually in the shape of a *T* or a 7. The frameless IUD (GyneFix) does away with the frame and consists of a small, free-floating thread anchored at one end.

Some IUDs are inert, others have and release copper, and some release a hormone—a progestin. The hormonal or hormone-releasing IUD is the one used to manage the menstrual period. Because of this we'll focus only on, and list only those characteristics that apply to, the hormone-releasing IUD group. At the time of this writing, only one brand of these is in use, and others are being developed.

The hormone-releasing IUD in use, Mirena Intrauterine System (IUS), is a framed device. Another new frame device and a frameless one are under development. Mirena has been available for over ten years in Europe, and in 2000 it finally became available in the United States.

Who Can Use the Hormone-Releasing IUD?

Before we go into details, recall that there are many types of IUDs. Because only the hormone-releasing one can be used for menstrual management, that's the one we'll be concentrating on here. Moreover, we're going to highlight the characteristics most pertinent to period control as opposed to birth control. The hormone-releasing IUD is particularly useful if you:

* *Don't want to or can't use other hormonal methods.* You can use a hormone-releasing IUD even if you can't tolerate or have contraindications to using other hormonal methods, like the birth control pill or implants. This is because this type of IUD releases a very small, localized amount of hormone. This, in turn, reduces the risk of generalized, body-wide side effects.

* *Are a smoker over the age of 35.*

* *Have just given birth or had a pregnancy termination (post-abortion).*

* *Are breastfeeding.*

* *Have a history of breast cancer.*

* *Have certain medical conditions.* If you have any of the following medical conditions, you can use the hormone-releasing IUD:

• Stroke or blood vessel diseases (cerebrovascular disease)
• Heart vessel disease (coronary artery disease)
• Complicated migraines
• Increased risk of blood clots and complications (thromboembolism)
• Vascular disease associated with diabetes or lupus
• Active liver disease and lipid disorders

Who Cannot Use the Hormone-Releasing IUD?

Most of the contraindications to IUD use have to do with sexual activity and sexually transmitted infections (STIs). Clearly, if you're not sexually active these restrictions don't apply to you. Don't use this method if you have any of the following conditions:

* **Known or suspected pregnancy.**

* **An allergy to any of the IUD's components.**

* **An infection of the genital organs.** If you have a sexually transmitted infection (STI) or pelvic inflammatory disease (PID) or genital actinomycosis (an infection) you should not use an IUD. Some examples of STI are: gonorrhea, chlamydia, and HIV (the virus that causes AIDS). In addition, if you had a postdelivery (postpartum endometritis) or posttermination (postabortion) infection in the past three months, you should use another method. Finally, if you have a cervical or vaginal infection, including bacterial vaginosis, you should wait until the treatment is completed before using an IUD.

* **A condition that increases your susceptibility to infections.** If you have a condition that makes you more vulnerable to infections caused by microorganisms you should not use IUDs. Some examples are: leukemia, acquired immune deficiency syndrome (AIDS), or intravenous drug use.

* **A high risk of acquiring STIs (you or your partner).** If you have multiple sexual partners, or if you have a partner who has multiple sexual partners, you should not use an IUD.

* **Known or suspected cancer of the genital tract, including abnormal genital bleeding or an abnormal Pap smear.**

* **A history of, or a condition that predisposes you to, ectopic pregnancy.** If you use the IUD for birth control, your risk of having an ectopic pregnancy is lower than that for the general population. However, if you do become pregnant while using it, that

pregnancy is more likely to be an ectopic one. Conditions that predispose someone to having an ectopic pregnancy are:

• Past history of an ectopic pregnancy
• A history of PID and STIs
• A history of fallopian tube surgery
• Age over 35 years old

* **A previously inserted IUD that has not yet been removed.**
* **A condition that results in a distortion of the uterine cavity or a narrowing of the cervical canal.**

Advantages of Using the Hormone-Releasing IUD

You can use the hormone-releasing IUD to manage your menstrual period. In terms of advantages, this method:

* *Significantly reduces blood loss.* For example, women with heavy, prolonged bleeding (menorrhagia) who used this method for three months had a 94 percent reduction of their blood loss.

* *Can be as effective as surgery.* The hormone-releasing IUD can be used as a possible alternative to hysterectomy (removal of the uterus), and one study found it almost as effective as endometrial ablation (a surgical procedure) at reducing bleeding over one to two years.

* *Acts locally, inside the uterine cavity, so widespread side effects are limited.* A major advantage of the hormone-releasing IUD over long-acting, systemic hormonal methods (like implants) is the fact that it acts locally, minimizing body-wide effects.

Additionally, the hormone-releasing IUD:

* *Can be used by women who don't want to, or can't, use other types of hormonal birth control methods.* Even if you cannot tolerate other progestin-only methods, like implants, you can use the hormone-releasing IUD because it releases a very small, localized amount of hormone.

* *Offers highly effective, long-term, immediately reversible protection against pregnancy.* The hormone-releasing IUD gives you better pregnancy protection than does "getting the tubes tied" (female sterilization): for the IUD the failure rate is 0.1 percent, while for the surgery it's 0.4 percent. For young women who have not had a child, an IUD is more effective than the Pill. (If you don't have children, please discuss with your physician if you are a good candidate for the IUD.) Also, this method is long-acting, it doesn't interfere with the spontaneity of sexual intercourse, and fertility returns immediately once the IUD is removed. (Pregnancy rates are not affected by the duration of IUD use.)

* *Lowers the risk of an ectopic pregnancy.* Women who use an IUD (the second-generation copper and the newer, hormone-releasing ones) are less likely to experience an ectopic pregnancy than are women using no birth control. However, remember that if you do become pregnant while using an IUD, that pregnancy is more likely to be an ectopic. For example, with Mirena, a study showed there was an incidence of 0.2 ectopic pregnancies per 1,000 woman-years.

* *Lowers the risk of infection.* The hormone-releasing IUD thickens the cervical mucus, thus making it potentially more difficult for the bacteria to get up into the uterus. Also, Mirena appears to reduce the risk of pelvic infections. However, this doesn't mean you should rely on the IUD to protect against PID or sexually transmitted infections (STIs). If you are sexually active, use a barrier method, like the condom, to reduce your risk of acquiring an STI.

Disadvantages of Using the Hormone-Releasing IUD

The particular disadvantages of the hormone-releasing IUD are:

* *Irregular, heavy bleeding or spotting for the first three to six months of use*

* *Increased incidence of noncancerous (functional) ovarian cysts*

* *Higher risk of ectopic pregnancy*

The other side effects of this type of IUD are the ones commonly seen with progestin use, such as breast discomfort, mood changes (very rare), and nausea (see page 146), and the ones associated with IUD use in general, such as the possibility that the device could slip out of the uterus (rare) or perforate of the uterus.

How Do You Use the Hormone-Releasing IUD?

This is how the IUD works: the hormone, which is impregnated in the frame, is slowly released, over years, and it acts almost exclusively in the uterus.

THE BIRTH CONTROL REGIMEN

Any IUD (whether it's a hormonal one or not) is placed inside the uterus by a medical professional during a regular office visit. It takes a couple of minutes to put the IUD in, and the procedure is usually painless, or at most slightly uncomfortable (crampy). The insertion is usually done within seven days from the start of the period, but it can be done at any time during the monthly cycle, or immediately after a pregnancy termination, or within six to eight weeks of a delivery. Once the IUD is in, it works for five years. You can have the IUD removed at any time, by a medical professional, also in a matter of minutes. Removing the IUD is painless; it shouldn't cause you any discomfort.

THE MENSTRUAL MANAGEMENT REGIMEN

The hormone-releasing IUD is a very good method to use if your period control goals are to:

* Significantly reduce the amount of blood flow

* Shorten the period's duration and even stop bleeding (amenorrhea) altogether

* Reduce, or even eliminate, painful periods

For example, this method will help if:

* You have a condition, such as anemia, uterine fibroids, or endometriosis, that can be made worst by having heavy periods.

* You're considering surgery for your period-related problems and would like to first try a less drastic option.

The same regimen used for birth control is used for menstrual management: the hormone-releasing IUD is inserted into the uterus and you keep it in place for as long as you want to or need to use it (up to five years).

There are several advantages to using the hormone-releasing IUD. Because the hormone in the IUD is released slowly over time and acts locally on the uterine lining, it has less impact on the bleeding pattern. For example, after the first three to six months of use, you are less likely to experience breakthrough bleeding and spotting; after the second year of use, about 30 to 50 percent of women no longer have any bleeding at all. Hormone-releasing IUDs are very useful for women who can't or do not want to use a hormonal method that has estrogen, or other progestin-only methods. They are also very good for women with period-related problems, like heavy periods, and/or health problems, like anemia, uterine fibroids, and endometriosis. Another group of women for whom the hormone-releasing IUD is ideally suited is women who are interested in period control as well as simultaneous, long-term birth control.

The main disadvantage of using the hormone-releasing IUD is that you can't regulate the bleeding pattern. For example, up to 50 percent of women using Mirena stop having periods altogether, but there's no way to predict in advance which women this will apply to.

The bottom line: if you're interested in active management and you're able to use estrogen, the IUD isn't the best option for you. However, for women who don't want to, or can't, use estrogen, the hormone-releasing IUD is a very good option. You can consider this method even if you're interested in relatively short-term (one year) period control, although using this method long-term is the better option.

About Specific Brands of Hormone-Releasing IUDs

Let's take a moment now to look at Mirena and two hormone-releasing IUDs under development.

MIRENA INTRAUTERINE SYSTEM (IUS)

The Mirena Intrauterine System (IUS) has a plastic, T-shaped frame that contains 52 milligrams of the progestin levonorgestrel in the vertical arm. The IUS gradually releases a very small amount of hormone every day (20 micrograms) and it can be used for five years. LevoNova is Mirena's counterpart in the Scandinavian countries. Mirena has been used in Europe for more than ten years, and in December 2000, it was also finally approved for use in the United States.

Mirena is especially useful for women with heavy, prolonged, or painful menstrual periods, because it:

* *Significantly reduces the monthly blood loss.* Approximately 90 percent of women who use Mirena have a reduction in their menstrual bleeding. In fact, this type of IUD can be used (off-label) as a possible alternative to hysterectomy (the surgical removal of the uterus) as a treatment for heavy menstrual bleeding. For example, the number of days of bleeding is re-

duced from seven days, during the first month of use, to two days, during the twelfth month. This is a very important benefit of using this IUD, considering that in the United States about 118,000 hysterectomies are performed annually for this reason alone.

* *Stops monthly bleeding*. After one year of using Mirena, up to 50 percent of women stop having a monthly bleeding episode altogether.

* *Reduces menstrual pain (dysmenorrhea)*. Because the hormone released by this IUD acts locally, inside the uterus, it greatly reduces the secretion of the substances (prostaglandins) that have a role in producing painful periods.

Mirena is also beneficial because it:

* *Reduces the bleeding associated with uterine fibroids*. For example, one study found that 95 percent of women with fibroids who were anemic and who used this method were no longer anemic after one year of use.

When it comes to menstrual management, the particular disadvantage associated with the use of Mirena is bleeding and spotting, sometimes heavy, mostly during the first three to six months of use.

Resource: http://www.mirena-us.com (site maintained by the manufacturer).

FEMILIS T
Currently being developed is Femilis T, a framed hormone-releasing IUD that releases 14 micrograms of the progestin levonorgestrel per day (compared to 20 micrograms per day for Mirena). The intended lifespan of this brand of IUD is ten years (compared to Mirena's five years). Femilis T will come in two models, one for women who have never had children (nulliparous), and one for those who already have given birth (parous).

The advantages of this IUD for menstrual management use are that it:

* *Releases less daily hormone and has a longer lifespan*
* *Should be easier to insert and retain*

The device is smaller and more flexible in order to allow for an easy insertion even in the small uteri of women who have never had children. Also, because the arms unfold immediately upon insertion of the IUD into the uterine cavity, the risk of perforation is likely to be reduced. The end result is that this model will likely have fewer troublesome side effects such as disturbed bleeding patterns, including amenorrhea, and hormonal side effects.

As with any hormone-releasing IUD in general, the main disadvantage is that, if you're interested in active period control, the hormone-releasing IUD wouldn't be your first choice.

This new type of IUD looks promising for women who suffer from heavy and painful periods, or other period-related medical problems, and who might not have been able to tolerate the available IUDs.

FIBROPLANT-LNG INTRAUTERINE SYSTEM (IUS)

A frameless IUD, as the name implies, is an IUD that doesn't have the rigid, or semiflexible, plastic frame seen in the framed brands. The frameless IUD currently in use is the GyneFix (and the GyneFix mini), which consists of six (four for the mini) small copper sleeves threaded on a suture string.

Using a frameless IUD has several advantages over using the regular framed IUD—better tolerated, less likelihood of expulsion. In addition, when it comes to the menstrual period, this type of IUD doesn't increase period bleeding and reduces cramping. When you use an inert (no copper, no hormone) IUD, like the Lippes Loop, your menstrual blood loss could be about twice (70–80 milliliters) that of a normal period due to the inert frame. With a copper IUD, like one of the copper T series, the amount of excess bleeding is less

(50–60 milliliters). In contrast, GyneFix, particularly the GyneFix mini, does not increase your menstrual blood loss (compared to the period prior to IUD use). Of course, a hormone-releasing IUD like Mirena actually decreases the amount of monthly blood loss. But, because Mirena has a frame, that in itself can cause spotting and cramping compared to a frameless IUD like GyneFix.

So developing a frameless, hormone-releasing IUD would be very helpful, because it would combine the best features of GyneFix (no frame, less cramping) and Mirena (hormone-releasing, less bleeding). Enter FibroPlant.

FibroPlant consists of a small rod (about 3 centimeters long), which houses the hormone and the conventional anchoring system used for frameless IUDs. The progestin levonorgestrel is released at a rate of 14 micrograms per day, for a period of three years. A version designed to last a minimum of five years is also under development.

The advantages of this type of IUD, for menstrual management use, are:

* *Reduced incidence of cramping and pain.* Because FibroPlant doesn't have a frame and it's shorter than the original frameless one (GyneFix), it tends to adapt very well to uterine cavities of various sizes and shapes. This greatly minimizing the discomfort/cramping and expulsion seen with the use of the framed IUDs. Also, because it releases hormone, which acts locally inside the uterus, it greatly reduces the secretion of prostaglandins, substances that have a role in causing painful periods (dysmenorrhea).

* *Significantly reduced amount of bleeding.* In women with regular but heavy menstrual bleeding and anemia, this method significantly reduces the amount of blood lost. For example, the reduction of menstrual blood loss is at least 80 percent and it occurs as early as one month after insertion.

* *Fewer disturbances in the bleeding pattern.* Because of the reduced dose of hormone released by this type of IUD, fewer

women experience breakthrough spotting or bleeding, and complete absence of monthly bleeding. Of course, some users might consider this a disadvantage. However, if you're a woman who wants or needs to use menstrual management, but prefers to have a monthly episode of bleeding, this is clearly an advantage for you.

The main disadvantage of the frameless hormone-releasing IUD is that you won't be able to use it for active menstrual management.

The frameless hormone-releasing IUD will be particularly useful for women who have tried to use an IUD but were unable to tolerate other types of IUDs in the past. It will also help women with heavy or painful periods and those with uterine fibroids.

So far, we've discussed the hormonal methods of birth control that can be used for active menstrual management (the combination pill, the skin patch, and the vaginal ring), as well as the ones that can be used for passive management (the progestin-only pill, the shot, the implant, and the hormone-releasing IUD). Of course, in addition to the regimens we touched upon, there are other regimens used to manage the period. These are mostly used for medical conditions—very heavy bleeding in an anemic woman—but can also be used for an unexpected, important life event, like an unscheduled performance or event for a professional artist or athlete. However, these regimens (high dose or multidose) involve using higher doses of estrogen and/or progestin than the ones we've discussed here, and their risk/benefit profile is also different (for example, nausea and vomiting tend to be more common). Your physician can discuss more details with you.

Surgery

In addition to all the medical methods we've discussed, another group of methods used for period control is the surgical one.

Before we proceed, we need to make one thing very clear. None of the surgical methods we'll mention here are dual use, like the hormonal birth control methods: none of the surgeries are or should be used as a method of birth control. Also, since any surgery is an invasive procedure, these methods are not intended for, nor are they to be used for, short-term lifestyle issues or minor period-related health problems. If you want to stop having periods for spring break or you want to regulate your periods, surgery on your uterus is not the way to go. Actually, in general, even for women for whom having a monthly period is detrimental to their health, it's always beneficial to first try to use one of the nonsurgical methods of period control. If it helps, great! Then there is no need to go on to surgery, and all risks associated with surgery are avoided. If it doesn't, you can proceed to the more invasive surgery step knowing that you've made an informed decision. So, as a rule, think of the surgical methods as the really big guns of menstrual management.

As an aside, a surgical method may not always be better than a medical one in the long run. Of course, this is all relative and depends on your particular circumstances and condition, so your personal physician is the best resource for your decision. The point is, make sure you're familiar with, and you explore, all the available options before considering using a surgical method.

So, let's now quickly review the surgeries connected with period control. This is a brief, noncomprehensive discussion and your physician will be able to describe all the benefits and risks, indications, and particulars of each procedure in detail.

Dilatation and Curettage (D&C)

Briefly, this surgical procedure involves dilatation of the cervical canal and scraping (curettage) of the lining of the uterus. Think of this as a surgical period. After the procedure, the lining of the uterus is very thin, so there'll be no bleeding for a while (until the next period). Once the lining regrows, the bleeding returns. That's the reason why a D&C, while good at stopping acute bleeding, is not usually first-line therapy. The risks of undergoing a surgical procedure could outweigh the benefits you derive from something that's not a long-term solution. Actually, the same result—stopping the acute bleeding—can be achieved using a high-dose/multidose estrogen, progestin, or combination estrogen/progestin hormone regimen.

Bottom line: when it comes to period control, a D&C is not the first line of treatment, but it's an option you should be aware of.

Endometrial Ablation

Endometrial ablation is a surgical procedure in which most of the lining of the uterine cavity is destroyed. In contrast to a D&C, in which a sharp surgical instrument is used to do the scraping, in an ablation various other methods, like heat (hydrothermal) or freezing (cryoablation), are used. This procedure is used to treat women who suffer from abnormal or problem uterine bleeding, like chronic heavy, prolonged periods. In general, after endometrial ablation, depending on the technique used, 50–75 percent of women stop having periods altogether or bleed much less than previously. However, over time it's possible for the period, and thus the problem, to return (in about 15–20 percent of cases). Once you've had this procedure, one thing that's most probably not going to return is your ability to become pregnant. So, for women who plan a future pregnancy, this is not the procedure to have.

This surgical procedure, which can reduce and/or eliminate periods, is best reserved for women who have completed their families and who want to undergo a less drastic procedure than a hysterectomy (see next section). Of course, endometrial ablation is not a birth control method.

Myomectomy, Hysterectomy, and Oophorectomy

Myomectomy means removal of a uterine fibroid. Because these fibroids often cause heavy, prolonged menstrual bleeding, women suffering from this problem will have relief after the surgery. The problem is that these fibroids tend to recur, and there's no way to predict in advance which women this will happen to. So, after having a myomectomy, it's quite possible you'll find yourself right back where you started, experiencing the same problem. (The usual recurrence rate after myomectomy is 25 percent.) An alternative to myomectomy is a procedure called *uterine artery embolization*. Briefly, this is a less invasive procedure in which, under radiological guidance, the vessel that supplies blood to the fibroid is blocked. Since the fibroid is deprived of needed blood supply, it stops growing and shrivels up.

Hysterectomy means removal of the uterus. There are about 590,000 hysterectomies performed each year in the United States; in 20 percent of the cases the reason for the surgery is problem uterine bleeding. *Oophorectomy* means removal of the ovary. Obviously, once either the uterus or both ovaries are removed, you no longer can or will have menstrual periods, nor will you be fertile. (If only one ovary is removed, both fertility and menstrual periods are retained.)

All three of the surgical procedures mentioned here—myomectomy, hysterectomy, and oophorectomy—are major surgical procedures. They can be performed abdominally (via a cut on the abdomen similar to the one for a Cesarean section), laparoscopically (via small puncture cuts, using fiberoptic instruments), or vaginally. Obviously, none of these surgeries are birth control methods. And, while myomectomy may be viewed as a surgical period control method, think of hysterectomy and oophorectomy as the ultimate period control methods. This doesn't mean that there aren't women who can't truly benefit from these major surgeries and for whom these surgeries are the only way to help them. Rather, it means that it's always prudent and in your best interest to explore all the available options before making a decision. Your physician will be able to walk you through all the steps, as well as describe the advantages and disadvantages, of having these surgeries and assist you in making the best decision for your particular circumstances.

Using Menstrual Management and Birth Control

Millions of women are sexually active and are using birth control. While the ideal birth control method—one that is 100 percent effective in preventing pregnancy and STIs, has no side effects, and can be used by anyone—hasn't been invented yet, women today have an array of methods to chose from. For example, there are seven groups of birth control with over forty subgroups, and over eighty individual methods. (See Appendix A.)

With all these methods to choose from, if you're a sexually active woman considering using menstrual management you might feel confused and overwhelmed. Not only do you have to weight the advantages and disadvantages of using period control, but you also have to worry how your current method of birth control will fit into the picture. The obvious easy way out would be for one to suggest that, since all the hormonal menstrual management options can also be used for pregnancy protection, you should simply give up your current method of birth control and start using one of the hormonal methods. However, that is a presumptuous suggestion. As the "Sponge worthy" episode of *Seinfeld* so realistically portrayed—Elaine finds out that the birth control sponge is being taken off the market and scours the city to buy out the remaining sponge stock; she then judges potential partners in terms of "Sponge-worthiness"—once you're fortunate enough to find the birth control best suited to your unique needs, changing it is just not something you're likely to be inclined to do.

Fortunately, when it comes to using birth control and period control at the same time, you have options. For most birth control methods, there's a convenient way to integrate using a menstrual management method without having to give up your current method of birth control. Unfortunately, it's impossible to cover all the possible individual permutations. For more details on using menstrual management and birth control at the same time, please talk to your health-care professional or visit www.tcoyp.com.

Chapter Six Bibliography

Cunningham GF, Grant NF, Leveno KJ, *et al*, eds. Oral progestins. In: *Williams Obstetrics*. 21st ed. New York, NY: McGraw-Hill; 2001: 1531–3.

Mishell DR. Helping a woman choose: evaluating metabolic issues of oral contraceptives. In: *Understanding Contraceptive Choices: The Patient's Perspective*. 2003 Nov:3–4.

Sulak PJ. Creative use of oral contraceptives: perimenopause, menstrual disorders, premenstrual syndrome, and extended regimens. In: *Understanding Contraceptive Choices: The Patient's Perspective*. 2003 Nov: 16–18.

Kjos SL, Peters RK, Xiang A, *et al*. Contraception and the risk of type 2 diabetes in Latina women with prior gestational diabetes. *JAMA*. 1998; 280:533–8.

Jamin C. Macroprogestative contraception: advantages. (Article in French.) *Contracept Fertil Sex* (Paris). 1993 Feb;21(2):123–8.

Kaunitz AM, Westhoff C, Leonhardt KK. Therapeutic options to reduce or halt menstruation. *Female Patient*. 2002 Apr;27(Suppl):S15.

Irvine GA, Campbell-Brown MB, Lumsden MA, *et al*. Randomised comparative trial of the levonorgestrel intrauterine system and norethisterone for treatment of idiopathic menorrhagia. *Br J Obstet Gynaecol*. 1998;105:592–8.

Cerazette. Prescribing information. Organon. July 1999.

Cunningham GF, Grant NF, Leveno KJ, *et al*, eds. Injectable progestin contraceptives. In: *Williams Obstetrics*. 21st ed. New York, NY: McGraw-Hill; 2001:1533–4.

Kaunitz AM, Westhoff C, Leonhardt KK. Therapeutic options to reduce or halt menstruation. *Female Patient*. 2002 Apr;27(Suppl): S14–15.

Speroff L. Bone mineral density and hormonal contraception. In: *Dialogues in Contraception*. Summer 2002;7(5):2–3.

Kaunitz AM, Wysocki SJ. Misperceptions about steriodal contraceptives and IUDs. In: *Dialogue in Contraception*. Winter 2002;7(7):2–3.

Cunningham GF, Grant NF, Leveno KJ, *et al*, eds. Injectable medroxyprogesterone acetate/estradiol cypionate. In: *Williams Obstetrics*. 21st ed. New York, NY: McGraw-Hill; 2001:1535.

Darney PD, Speroff L. New methods. In: *Dialogues in Contraception*. Winter 2001;7(3):1.

Fraser IS. Vaginal bleeding patterns in women using once-a-month injectable contraceptives. *Contraception*. 1994;49(4);399–420.

Cunningham GF, Grant NF, Leveno KJ, *et al*, eds. Progestin implants (Norplant system). In: *Williams Obstetrics*. 21st ed. New York, NY: McGraw-Hill; 2001: 1534–5.

Darney PD. Contraceptive implants update. In: *Dialogues in Contraception*. Winter 2001;7(3):4.

Croxatto HB. Clinical profile of Implanon: a single-rod etonogestrel contraceptive implant. *Eur J Contracept Reprod Health Care*. 2000 Sep;5 (Suppl 2):21–8.

Cunningham GF, Grant NF, Leveno KJ, *et al*, eds. Failure and continuation rates at one year for various methods of birth control. In: *Williams Obstetrics*. 21st ed. New York, NY: McGraw-Hill; 2001:1520–1538.

Why are women not using long-acting contraceptives? In: *Ob/Gyn Clinical Alert*. Oct 2000;17(6):41–3.

Makarainen L, van Beek A, Tuomivaara L, *et al*. Ovarian function during the use of a single contraceptive implant: Implanon compared with Norplant. *Fertil Steril*. 1998 Apr;69(4):714–21.

Cox ML. The Dalkon Shield saga. *J Fam Planning Repro Health Care*. 2003;29(1):8.

Grimes DA. IUD safety. In: *Dialogues in Contraception*. Summer 2001; 7(1):4.

Farley TMM, Rosenberg MJ, Row PJ, *et al*. Intrauterine devices and pelvic inflammatory disease: an international perspective. *Lancet*. 1992;339: 785–8.

Mishell DR Jr., Bell JH, Good RG, *et al*. The intrauterine device: A bacteriologic study of the endometrial cavity. *Am J Obstet Gynecol*. 1966; 96:119–26.

American College of Obstetricians and Gynecologists (ACOG). National survey of women obstetricians/gynecologists. Gallup Survey, September 2003.

Cunningham GF, Grant NF, Leveno KJ, *et al*, eds. Intrauterine contraceptive devices. In: *Williams Obstetrics*. 21st ed. New York, NY: McGraw-Hill; 2001:1535–41.

Lahteenmaki P, Haukkamaa M, Puolakka J, *et al*. Open randomised study of use of levonorgestrel releasing intrauterine system as alternative to hysterectomy. *BMJ*. 1998; 316(7138):1122–6.

Romer T. Prospective comparison study of levonorgestrel IUD versus roller-ball endometrial ablation in the management of refractory recurrent hypermenorrhea. *Eur J Obstet Gynecol Repro Biol.* 2000;90:27–9.

Sivin I, Stern J. Health during prolonged use of levonorgestrel 20 mcg/d and the Copper TCu 380Ag intrauterine contraceptive devices: A multicenter study. International Committee for Contraception Research (ICCR). *Fertil Steril.* 1994;61:70–7.

Hidalgo M, Bahamondes L, Perrotti M, *et al.* Bleeding patterns and clinical performance of the levonorgestrel-releasing intrauterine system (Mirena) up to two years. *Contraception.* 2002;65(2):129–32.

Andersson K, Odlind V, Rybo G. Levonorgestrel-releasing and copper-releasing (Nova T) IUDs during five years of use: a randomized comparative trial. *Contraception.* 1994;49:56–72.

Burkman RT, Miller L. Extended and continuous use of hormonal contraceptives. In: *Dialogues in Contraception.* Winter 2004;8(4):3.

Monteiro I, Bahamondes L, Diaz J, *et al.* Therapeutic use of levonorgestrel-releasing intrauterine system in women with menorrhagia: a pilot study. *Contraception.* May 2002;65(5):325–8.

Hubacher D, Grimes DA. Noncontraceptive health benefits of intrauterine devices: a systematic review. *Obstet Gynecol Surv.* 2002 Feb;57(2): 120–8.

Wildemeersch D, Dhont M, Weyers S, *et al.* Miniature long-term intrauterine drug delivery for more effective contraception in adolescents. Florence presentation. 2–5 December 2002. (E-mail communication, Dr. Dirk Wildemeersch.)

Wildemeersch D. Miniature, low-dose, intrauterine drug delivery systems. *5th Athens Congress on Women's Health and Disease lecture.* 26–29 Sept 2002. Athens, Greece.

Wildemeersch D, Van Kets H, Vrijens M, *et al.* Intrauterine contraception in adolescent women. The GyneFix intrauterine implant. *Ann NY Acad Sci.* 1997 Jun 17;816:440–50.

Wildemeersch D, Schacht E, Wildemeersch P. Contraception and treatment in the perimenopause with a novel "frameless" intrauterine levonorgestrel-releasing drug delivery system: an extended pilot study. *Contraception.* 2002 Aug;66(2):93–9.

Conclusion

* * *

When it comes to information about the menstrual period and its management, it's very easy to feel confused and overwhelmed. You practically have to mount an expedition to find out the facts. And once you manage to gather all the needed information, you realize that everybody from your aunt Georgina to a multi-titled TV expert has period-related advice. All this is enough to discourage even the most determined women.

To choose an option that's beneficial to your needs, it's not enough to have the information; you have to be able to evaluate it. The good news is you can do that by following a few simple steps. Obviously, your health-care professional is an invaluable resource. But the more information you have, and the better you're able to evaluate the information yourself, the better your particular needs will be met. After all, you know yourself best.

How Do You Decide if Menstrual Management Can Benefit You?

Managing their periods helps millions of women—blushing brides and teenagers, mailcarriers and CEOs, stay-at-home mothers, and even ballerinas, soldiers, and nuns. Which is all great and useful . . . to them. But, naturally, the important question is: How can you decide if menstrual management will benefit you? The answer lies in you taking a little time to learn about menstrual management—which you've already done by reading this book—and committing to become an active participant in decisions that affect you.

Here's a quick, practical way to make the most use of the information found in this book and formulate a plan of action. When it comes to menstrual management, you have two choices: to use it or not to use it. (Remember, the reason to use period control is to benefit you.) Understanding how menstrual management works allows you to identify and base your choice on the particular criteria important to your lifestyle and health. Armed with this data, and in consultation with your physician, you can be confident that you will make the best choice for you.

First, you need to decide if either your lifestyle or health can benefit from using menstrual management. If, after a careful and informed consideration, your answer is no, then you're done. Clearly, in your judgment, period control is not for you. On the other hand, if you think period control will benefit you, you need to move to the next step: identifying your unique criteria for using this tool. For example, when considering whether to use period control, your criteria might include preparing for an upcoming event, relieving problems with your period, dealing with lifestyle or health issues, and/or attaining ongoing pregnancy protection. Because the criteria you use are unique to you, it's possible for two women in similar situations to reach opposite decisions about using period control. Moreover, your criteria will most likely change over time. When they do, it's time to re-evaluate your decision about using menstrual management.

For now, let's assume you've identified one or several criteria. The third step is to evaluate the impact of each of the two choices— to use or not to use menstrual management—on your criteria. In other words, once you have your reasons you need to do a "cost/benefit" analysis. Of course, this evaluation will encompass many aspects—when should you start using it, for how long, how will it impact your health, which method should you use, what are the costs involved—and the assistance of your physician or health-care provider is essential. But once you're able to identify what's important to you and why, most of the hard work is done.

Being able to judge the quality of medical information is also very important and can be very helpful to you when you formulate a plan of action. Reviewing a few of the basic concepts of evaluating and critiquing medical data should help make the task of judging information about period control a lot easier. Let's first look at a few pointers on how to evaluate medical information, and then briefly touch on how you can assess the merits of medical criticism.

Evaluating Medical Information

Medical information can perplex even seasoned scientists. Because medical studies involve human subjects, they can be difficult to devise and carry out; the methodology is often complex; and, last but not least, it's relatively easy to manipulate the results or to use the data out of context.

Evaluating the quality of medical information and studies is not an easy task, even for health-care professionals. But we get help. Medical journals usually present a study followed immediately by an expert critique that evaluates the strengths and weakness of the study, and comments, with evidence, on its conclusion. Unfortunately, nonmedical people don't get a lot of assistance. When it comes to health news, the media seem to enjoy preying on fears. Any health information sound byte or headline that might boost ratings tends to get wide exposure. It's important for you to be able to evaluate, at least at a basic level, the medical studies and information on which you'll base your lifestyle and health decisions. So, short of hiring your own personal medical expert to assist you, what can you do maximize your ability to assess health information? Here are a few practical tips that should help in your evaluation:

1) DON'T COMPARE APPLES AND ORANGES.

When you evaluate medical information, judge the evidence on its scientific merits and nothing else. Evaluate its medical validity, not its social, cultural, or political aspects. For example, say a male scientist is the author of a study that concludes that monthly periods are not the biological norm. While it's true that women have been underrepresented in authoring medical studies and have been oppressed for centuries, and that some men consider women inferior, none of these are relevant criteria for evaluating the study. If you're trying to find out what percentage of period-related articles are written by women, the author's gender is central to your evaluation of the study. If, however, you're trying to find out what the biological norm for periods is, the author's gender is irrelevant.*

2) BE VIGILANT.

Always watch for bias and manipulation. These are two common problems, and they can each affect the value of the information you're evaluating. Various types of bias (selection, detection bias) are inherent in medical studies. Good studies make an effort to minimize bias. Not only that, but in medical circles, for a study to be considered acceptable it has to point out its biases and weakness. The problem is that the nightly news or newspapers rarely cover an issue in-depth enough to even mention a study's bias.

Unfortunately, medical information is often manipulated in order to support a favorite position or predetermined conclusion. Sometimes this is due to ignorance; other times it is intentional. Here's a

---

*Note: In our example, the only time it would be relevant to consider nonmedical factors like the author's gender or personal beliefs would be if they are used as criteria in the study. For example, if the author of the study said it's not natural for woman to have monthly periods because men are superior to women, or because the Goddess of Menstruation said so, nonmedical factors may certainly be affecting the validity of the study.

sample headline I made up: *What You Don't Know Could Kill You: Use the Pill, Triple Your Risk of Blood Clot Problems!* It's true that a lack of information could kill you; it's also true that if you take the Pill your risk of developing a serious side effect related to blood clots (venous thromboembolism [VTE]) is increased threefold, compared to a woman who doesn't use the Pill. What the headline doesn't mention is that, even with this increase, the risk of VTE is still extremely low: 1 to 3 per 10,000 woman-years. That's because the VTE risk in this general population is very small to begin with: 1 in 10,000 woman-years. One other essential piece of information the headline omits: pregnant women have the highest risk of VTE—5.7 per 10,000 woman-years. Here's an equally true variant of my original headline: *You're More Likely to Die from Accidental Poisoning or a Car Accident than from a Blood Clot Problem.* That's how manipulation works.

3) CONSIDER THE SOURCE.

Always keep in mind that not all studies are created equal. Certain types of studies, because of the way they are designed and carried out, provide more useful information than others. A theory isn't a study. You shouldn't base health decisions on theories.

There are several types of medical studies (cross-over, cohort) and each has its strengths and weaknesses. The evidence from some is better than that from others. In general, assuming that the study is properly set up and conducted, here is a hierarchy of study types, from the ones with the best (strongest) evidence, to the ones with the weakest evidence:

1. EXPERIMENTAL STUDIES:
  a) Randomized Controlled Clinical Trial
  b) Randomized Cross-Over Clinical Trial
  c) Randomized Controlled Laboratory Study

These are the studies that can establish a cause-effect relationship. Why is this important? Because other types of studies, like the epidemiological studies that you see most often speculated in the media, only establish an association between a *presumed* cause and an effect. This is hardly, if ever, pointed out in the media.

2. OBSERVATIONAL STUDIES:
   a) Cohort
   b) Case-Control
   c) Ecologic (Aggregate)
   d) Cross-Sectional
   e) Case Series
   f) Case Report*

*Imagine I had included twenty personal testimonials from women, describing their wonderful experience with using the Pill for menstrual management. An entertaining and emotionally rich read, for sure. Yet, at the same time, completely irrelevant as useful medical information. I, as a physician, can't make any recommendation based on the letters. Likewise, you can't use the information to make informed decisions about what to do. That's not because the women's experience or opinions are worthless; rather, because of all the variables involved, an individual case provides little useful empirical evidence. Because a case report is nothing more than a personal experience observed and reported by a physician, the evidence it provides is limited. When it comes to what's best for you, nothing beats objective medical evidence.

Finally, let's use an example to illustrate how you can critique the critics. This is not a valid medical criticism of a study that says the monthly period is unnatural:

"The silly, greedy, and funny-looking author of the study says, oh horror of horrors, that monthly periods are unnatural. Because this means the author is 'anti-period' and is saying that the monthly period is an ailment, this study is worthless and an attempt to subjugate women and enrich a nefarious group of conspirators hiding in the forest (and I also hope a house falls on this author)."

On the other hand, this is:

"The author says that monthly menstrual periods are unnatural. This means the author is saying that the monthly period is an ailment because of facts, a, b, and c. Since facts a, b, and c are incorrect, because x, y, and z, the author's assertion that menstrual periods are unnatural is incorrect. Thus the entire study is incorrect."

Bottom line: Be suspicious when you see emotional or inflammatory terms used. Chances are the material represents a personal point of view rather than useful facts. While personal opinions can be good for our ego, they're not very helpful when it comes to making informed health decisions. Medical facts are neutral—they're neither good nor bad—and medical discussions, even criticism, should be free of personal viewpoints and bombast.

Red flags should go up when you see a lot of unrelated and unsubstantiated claims. Valid medical criticism addresses relevant information and offers supporting evidence. Valid criticism uses neutral language, states the accepted facts, and points out, again in a neutral tone, what the potential concern might be. It helps you with your decision because it teaches you.

Just as I was preparing to write the conclusion for this book, I noticed a commercial on TV about a relatively new birth control pill brand, *Yasmin*. As the female voice-over mentioned that this pill can also help you with problems you might have "during that time of the month," I had two simultaneous reactions: I thought it's great that we can finally have some information on TV about birth control (among all the beer and impotence adds), and I shouted at the TV, *"Call it by name—the menstrual period, or the period!"*

Despite all the great developments in our society, and all the progress made, there's still a reluctance to entrust women with making responsible decisions. No matter who you are or what you do, you have responsibilities and much is expected of you. Yet hardly an eyebrow is raised when, almost at every turn, women are treated as if they are incapable of making decisions that will impact their lifestyle and health. It's considered perfectly acceptable to have nonmedical people regulate, influence, and have a say in medical matters, as long as the patient concerned is a woman. The debate seems always to be about who has women's best interests at heart and who's more heroic in protecting their interests; it's never about simply giving women the facts, and just the facts, and allowing them to decide.

In my opinion, the best way to end this practical guide to menstrual management is by offering you one final piece of parting advice: Trust yourself! It doesn't matter if you're a teenager still in school or a person in your forties with enough diplomas to wallpaper a room; an atheist stay-at-home mom or a religious astronaut; a libertarian rancher or an independent big-city civic leader. There's no reason why you, in consultation with your physician, can't make an informed decision or shouldn't have enough confidence in yourself and your abilities. All you need is a few tools—the basic information and an ability to evaluate it—and a desire to become an active participant in your own life. Granted, nothing worthwhile comes without an effort. Getting involved means assuming responsibility. But responsibility is equally worthwhile and brings rewards. Taking charge and getting involved empowers you to take advantage of the benefits afforded by having a voice in decisions that affect your life and your health and it also allows you to share your knowledge with other women. Always remember:

Knowledge will forever govern ignorance: And a people who mean to be their own governors, must arm themselves with the power knowledge gives.
>   —James Madison
>   4th President of the United States (1751–1836)

Appendix A

Birth Control Brands

* * *

MONOPHASIC BRANDS

Brand Name	Hormone Content Estrogen mg + Progestin mg (EE = Ethinyl Estradiol)
Demulen 1/50 Nelulen 1/50 Zovia 1/50	EE 0.05 + Ethynodiol diacetate 1.0
Neogynon 21 Nordiol 21 or 28 Ovran Stediril-D Tetragynon	EE 0.05 + Levonorgestrel 0.25
Gravistat Microgynon 50 Neo-Stediril	EE 0.05 + Levonorgestrel 0.125

Brand Name	Hormone Content Estrogen mg + Progestin mg (EE = Ethinyl Estradiol)
Ovostat	EE 0.05 + Lynestrenol 1.0
Ovcon 50	EE 0.05 + Norethindrone* 1.0
Milli-Anovlar *Norlestrin 1/50*	EE 0.05 + Norethindrone acetate 1.0
Norlestrin 2.5/50	EE 0.05 + Norethindrone acetate 2.5
Ovral *Ogestrel* *Stediril*	EE 0.05 + Norgestrel 0.5
Planor	EE 0.05 + Norgestrienone 2.0
Genora 1/50 *Necon 1/50* *Nelova 1/50M* *Norinyl 1/50* *Norethin 1/50M* *Ortho-Novum 1/50*	Mestranol 0.05 + Norethindrone 1.0
Yermonil	EE 0.04 + Lynestrenol 2
Ovoresta M *Ovostat micro*	EE 0.0375 + Lynestrenol 0.75
Brenda-35 *Diane-35* *Dianette*	EE 0.035 + Cyproterone acetate 2.0
Demulen 1/35 *Zovia 1/35*	EE 0.035 + Ethynodiol diacetate 1.0

*Norethindrone is also called norethisterone.

Brand Name	Hormone Content Estrogen mg + Progestin mg (EE = Ethinyl Estradiol)
GenCept 1/35 Genora 1/35 Necon 1/35 NEE 1/35 Nelova 1/35E Norcept-E 1/35 Norethin 1/35E Norimin Norinyl 1/35 Ortho-Novum 1/35 Ovysmen 1/35	EE 0.035 + Norethindrone 1.0
Brevicon Brevinor Modicon Necon 0.5/35 NEE 0.5/35 Nelova 0.5/35E Ovysmen 0.5/35	EE 0.035 + Norethindrone 0.5
Ovcon 35	EE 0.035 + Norethindrone 0.4
Cilest Effiprev Ortho-Cyclen	EE 0.035 + Norgestimate 0.25
Cycleane 30 Desogen Marvelon Ortho-Cept Varnoline	EE 0.03 + Desogestrel 0.15

Brand Name	Hormone Content Estrogen mg + Progestin mg (EE = Ethinyl Estradiol)
Femodene *Femodene ED* *Gynera* *Minulet* *Moneva*	EE 0.03 + Gestodene 0.075
Eugynon 30 *Ovran 30*	EE 0.03 + Levonorgestrel 0.25
Femigoa *Femranette*	EE 0.03 + Levonorgestrel 0.15
Levlen *Levora 0.15/30* *Microgynon 30* *Microgynon 30 ED* *Minidril* *Monofeme 28* *Nordette* *Ologyn micro* *Ovranette* *Seasonale*** *Stediril 30*	EE 0.03 + Levonorgestrel 0.15
Necon 0.5/30	EE 0.03 + Norethindrone 0.5
Loestrin 1.5/30	EE 0.03 + Norethindrone acetate 1.5
Lo-Ovral *Low-Ogestrel*	EE 0.03 + Norgestrel 0.3
Petibelle *Yasmin*	EE 0.03 + Drospirenone 3.0

**Seasonale is the only FDA-approved menstrual management–labeled brand.

Brand Name	Hormone Content Estrogen mg + Progestin mg (EE = Ethinyl Estradiol)
Nelulen 1/25	EE 0.025 + Ethynodiol diacetate 1.0
Necon 1/25	EE 0.025 + Norethindrone 1.0
Cycleane 20 *Mercilon*	EE 0.02 + Desogestrel 0.15
Femodette *Harmonet* *Meliane* *Meloden 21*	EE 0.02 + Gestodene 0.075
Alesse *Levlite* *Loette* *Microgynon 20 ED* *Miranova*	EE 0.02 + Levonorgestrel 0.10
Loestrin 1/20	EE 0.02 + Norethindrone acetate 1.0
Melodene 15 *Melodia* *Minesse‡* *Mirelle*	EE 0.015 + Gestodene 0.06

BIPHASIC BRANDS

Brand Name	Hormone Content Estrogen mg + Progestin mg (EE = Ethinyl Estradiol)
Gracial	EE 0.04 + Desogestrel 0.025 (7 days)/ EE 0.03 + Desogestrel 0.125 (15 days)

‡ Reduces the placebo interval from 7 to 4 days.

Brand Name	Hormone Content Estrogen mg + Progestin mg (EE = Ethinyl Estradiol)
Binordiol *Biphasil 28* *Sequilar ED*	EE 0.05 + Levonorgestrel 0.05 (11 days)/ EE 0.05 + Levonorgestrel 0.125 (10 days)
Physiostat*	EE 0.05 (7 days)/ EE 0.05 + Lynestrenol 1.0 (15 days)
Ovanon*	EE 0.05 (7 days)/ EE 0.05 + Lynestrenol 2.5 (15 days)
Jenest-28 *Necon 10/11* *NEE 10/11* *Nelova 10/11* *Ortho-Novum 10/11*	EE 0.035 + Norethindrone** 0.5 (10 days)/ EE 0.035 + Norethindrone 1.0 (11 days)
BiNovum	EE 0.035 + Norethisterone 0.5 (7 days)/ EE 0.035 + Norethisterone 1.0 (14 days)
Adepal	EE 0.03 + Levonorgestrel 0.15 (7 days)/ EE 0.04 + Levonorgestrel 0.2 (14 days)
Miniphase	EE 0.03 + Norethisterone acetate 1.0 (11 days)/ EE 0.04 + Norethisterone acetate 2.0 (10 days)
Mircette†	EE 0.02 + Desogestrel 0.15 (21 days)/ EE 0.01 (5 days)

*Sequential brand.

**Norethindrone is also called norethisterone.

† Has two placebo (inert) pills for days 22–23, and five pills containing EE 0.01 mg for days 24–28.

TRIPHASIC BRANDS

Brand Name	Hormone Content Estrogen mg + Progestin mg (EE = Ethinyl Estradiol)
Cyclessa	EE 0.025 + Desogestrel 0.1 (7 days)/ EE 0.025 + Desogestrel 0.125 (7 days)/ EE 0.025 + Desogestrel 0.15 (7 days)
Milvane *Phaeva* *Triadene* *TriMinulet* *Triodeen* *Trioden*	EE 0.03 + Gestodene 0.05 (6 days)/ EE 0.04 + Gestodene 0.07 (5 days)/ EE 0.03 + Gestodene 0.1 (10 days)
Logynon *Logynon ED* *NovaStep* *Trietti* *Trifeme* *Trigynon* *Tri-Levlen* *Trinordiol 21 and 28* *Trioga* *Triphasil* *Triquilar* *Trivora*	EE 0.03 + Levonorgestrel 0.05 (6 days)/ EE 0.04 + Levonorgestrel 0.075 (5 days)/ EE 0.03 + Levonorgestrel 0.125 (10 days)
Ortho-Novum 7/7/7	EE 0.035 + Norethindrone* 0.5 (7 days)/ EE 0.035 + Norethindrone 0.75 (9 days)/ EE 0.035 + Norethindrone 1.0 (5 days)
Synphasic *Tri-Norinyl*	EE 0.035 + Norethindrone 0.5 (7 days)/ EE 0.035 + Norethindrone 1.0 (9 days)/ EE 0.035 + Norethindrone 0.5 (5 days)

*Norethindrone is also called norethisterone.

Brand Name	Hormone Content Estrogen mg + Progestin mg (EE = Ethinyl Estradiol)
Estrostep	EE 0.020 + Norethindrone acetate 1.0 (5 days)/ EE 0.030 + Norethindrone acetate 1.0 (7 days)/ EE 0.035 + Norethindrone acetate 1.0 (9 days)
Triella *TriNovum*	EE 0.035 + Norethisterone* 0.5 (7 days)/ EE 0.035 + Norethisterone 0.75 (7 days)/ EE 0.035 + Norethisterone 1.0 (7 days)
Ortho Tri-Cyclen *Ortho Tri-Cyclen low* (EE 0.025)	EE 0.035 + Norgestimate 0.18 (7 days)/ EE 0.035 + Norgestimate 0.215 (7 days)/ EE 0.035 + Norgestimate 0.25 (7 days)

Progestin-Only Birth Control Pill

PROGESTIN-ONLY MINI-DOSE BRANDS

Brand Name	Progestin (mg)
Cerazette	Desogestrel 0.075
Femulen	Ethynodiol diacetate 0.5
Microlut (35) *Microval (35)* *Norgeston (35)*	Levonorgestrel 0.03
Exluton (28)	Lynestrenol 0.5
Locilan (28) *Micronor* *Micronovum (35)* *Noriday* *Nor-QD*	Norethisterone 0.35

*Norethistherone is also called norethindrone.

Brand Name	Progestin (mg)
Milligynon	Norethisterone* acetate 0.6
Neogest (35) *Ovrette*	Norgestrel 0.075
Ogyline	Norgestrienone 0.35

PROGESTIN-ONLY FULL-DOSE BRANDS

Brand Name	Progestin (mg)
Orgametril	Lynestrenol 5.0
Primolut-Nor	Norethisterone acetate 5.0
Lutéran	Chlormadinone acetate 10.0
Lutényl	Nomegestrol acetate 5.0
Surgestone	Promegestone 0.5

Shots

COMBINATION SHOT BRANDS

Brand Name	Estrogen (mg)	Progestin (mg)
Lunelle *Cyclofem* *Cyclofemina* *Novafem* *Cyclogestone*	Estradiol cypionate 5.0	Medroxyprogesterone acetate 25.0
Mesigyna *Norigynon*	Estradiol valerate 5.0	Norethisterone enanthate 50.0

*Norethisterone is also called norethindrone.

Brand Name	Estrogen (mg)	Progestin (mg)
Deladroxate* Perlutal (Perlutan) Unalmes Agurin Topasel Horprotal Uno-Ciclo	Estradiol enanthate 10.0	Dihydroxyprogesterone acetophenide 150.0
Yectames Anafertin	Estradiol enanthate 5.0	Dihydroxyprogesterone acetophenide 75.0
Chinese injectable No. 1	Estradiol valerate 5.0	17α-hydroxyprogesterone caproate 250.0

*Withdrawn.

Appendix B

Birth Control Groups

* * *

BIRTH CONTROL GROUPS

1. Hormonal
2. Nonsteroidal Pill
3. Intrauterine Devices (IUDs)
4. Barrier and Spermicide
5. Natural Family Planning
6. Sterilization
7. Emergency Contraception

1. Hormonal Group

- Pill
- Skin patch
- Vaginal ring
- Implants
- Shots (Injections)
- Hormone-releasing IUDs

2. Nonsteroidal Pill Group

- Centchroman

3. Intrauterine Device (IUD) Group

- Older IUDs
- Frame IUDs:
- First generation
- Second generation
- Newer IUDs
- Frameless IUD
- Hormone-releasing IUDs

4. **Barrier and Spermicide Group**
   - Male, female, and unisex condoms
   - Diaphragms:
     - Latex
     - Silicone
   - Cervical cap (Prentif, Vimule, Dumas, FemCap, Ovès)
   - Lea contraceptive (Lea's shield)
   - Sponges (Pharmatex, Today, Protectaid)
   - Spermicides (foam, cream, gel, jelly, suppository, film)

5. **Natural Family Planning Group**
   - Continuous abstinence
   - Outercourse
   - Sexual techniques:
     - Coitus interruptus (withdrawl)
     - Coitus reservatus
     - Coitus obstructus
   - Breastfeeding (lactational amenorrhea)
   - Fertility awareness (periodic abstinence):
     - Calendar
       - Rhythm (Ogino-Knaus)
       - Standard Days method (SDM)
       - CycleBeads
   - Basal Body Temperature (BBT)
     - BioSelf 110
     - Mini-Sofia
     - LadyComp
     - BabyComp
     - Cyclotest-2
   - Ovulation
     - Billings method
     - Creighton model
     - TwoDay method
   - Cervical changes
   - Sympto-Thermal methods
   - Personal hormone monitoring (Persona)

6. **Sterilization Group**
   - Male sterilization (vasectomy):
     - Conventional
     - No-scalpel
   - Female sterilization ("getting the tubes tied"):
     - Abdominal
   - Vaginal
   - Transcervical
     - Plugs (Essure pbc, Ovabloc, Hamou, P-block)
     - Chemical plugs
     - Quinacrine

7. **Emergency Contraception Group**
   - Combination pill
   - Progestin-only pill
   - Intrauterine devices (IUDs)
   - Antiprogesterone pill (Mifepristone or RU-486)
   - Progesterone production blocker pill (Epostane)

Index

* * *

Page numbers in *italic* indicate illustrations; those in **bold** indicate tables.

Three-phase (triphasic) cycle, Pill, 24, 154, **246–247**
Thromboembolic disease, 180, 192, 214
Timing of periods, 6
Toxic shock syndrome (TSS), 19, 20
Transvaginal route, 170
Triphasic (three-phase) cycle, Pill, 24, 154, **246–247**
Trophoblastic disease, 182
Trophoblast invasion, 65
TSS (toxic shock syndrome), 19, 20
Tuberculosis, 192
Tube tying (sterilization), **38**, 117, 217
Two-hormone shots, 190, 200–201
Two-phase (biphasic) cycle, Pill, 24, 153–154, **245–246**

U
UNICAMP University School of Medicine, 111
University of Washington School of Medicine, 121
Unnatural, monthly period as, 73–75
"Untouchable" menstruating women, 10, 16–17
Upper female genital tract, 38–45, *39. See also* Menstrual cycle; Uterus
  birth control methods and, **38**
  breast cancer and ovarian cysts, 39–40
  cervix, 41, 45
  corpus albicans (white body), 39, 59, 64
  corpus luteum (yellow body, CL), 39, 49, 58, 59, 62, *64*
  ectopic pregnancy, 44
  endometriosis, 42–43
  endometrium, 41, 62, 63
  fallopian tubes (uterine tubes, oviducts), 38, **38**, *39*, 41, 43–44, 57, 63
  fibroids (leiomyomas, myomas), 10, 12, 42
  intrauterine devices (IUDs), **38**
  myometrium, 42
  noncancerous (benign) ovarian tumors, 40, 143, 181, 184
  ostium, 41
  ova (eggs), 37, 38–39, 41, 57
  ovarian cysts, 39–40, 131
  ovaries, 37, **38**, 38–40, *39*, 41

pelvic inflammatory disease (PID), 19, 44–45
Pill, **39**
polycystic ovarian syndrome (PCOS), 40, 51
"retrograde flow" theory of endometriosis, 43
sexually transmitted infections (STIs), 44, 45
User profiles
  implants, 180–182, 203
  intrauterine devices (IUDs), 182, 214–216
  Pill, 139–141, 147
  progestin-only pill (POP), 180–182
  shots, 139–141, 147, 191–193
  skin patch (Ortho Evra), 139–141, 147, 163–164
  surgical methods of menstrual management, 224
  vaginal ring (NuvaRing), 139–141, 147, 168
Uterine artery embolization, 227
Uterine cancer
  fake periods, 111–112
  fat tissue and, 109
  menstrual management, 22, 181, 183
  myths about, 76
  Pill, 131, 143
  progestin-only pill (POP), 181, 183
  shots, 194
Uterine cycle (endometria, menstrual cycle), 56, 59–60, 62–64, *64*
Uterine fibroids
  intrauterine devices (IUDs), 219, 221, 224
  menstrual cycle, 42
  menstrual management, 10, 12
  Pill, 142–143
Uterine infections, 45, 66
Uterine tubes (fallopian tubes), 38, **38**, *39*, 41, 43–44, 57, 63
Uterus
  menstrual cycle, 36–37, 38, **38**, *39*, 40–45, 63
  myths about, 83–86

V
Vagina, 37, 38, **38**, 41, *46*, 46–47
Vaginal bulb, 47